Last Call

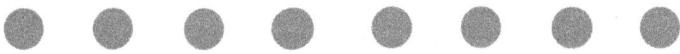

GAIL MITCAVISH

LAST CALL
© 2021 Gail Mitcavish

ISBNs:
Paperback: 979-8-9852695-0-5
eBook: 979-8-9852695-1-2

Edited by Elizabeth Garrett, Polished Printing
Designed by Mary Susan Oleson, Blu Design Concepts
Beer Mug photograph: Marco Verch
Printed in the U. S. A.

Chapter One

"BUT I'M LEAVING for the Betty Ford Center in the morning," I protested, struggling to gain hold of my thoughts as the judge sentenced me to three days in the Ottawa County Jail.

Handcuffs locked my wrists together when Judge Jones, responded, "Apparently you will not leave for Betty Ford in the morning, will you, Gail?"

I was led out of the courtroom, softly mumbling to myself—*how am I going to survive three days without alcohol and pills?*

Suffering in silence, my mind drifted back several weeks to the night I was arrested for my driving under the influence (DUI) on November 7, 1998. I planned on spending the night with my boyfriend, James, at his house for the weekend. However, after frantically clawing through my purse, I realized my bottle of pills was in the top drawer of my dresser in my bedroom. I only had three pills with me. A good addict always has an ample supply of pills in her pockets. It was my unwritten law. My pills of choice were Vicodin and Ativan. The first is a narcotic pain medication, and Ativan is prescribed for anxiety. Both are very addictive medications. Only for a moment I wondered if three pills would hold me over the weekend. I made my choice. I had to go out, and yet, I knew I shouldn't go. I was well into my second beer within a half hour…I don't remember the excuse (lie) I gave James. I do remember grabbing a beer from the fridge for my twenty-minute drive home.

I had scarcely driven one mile when I kinda, sorta ran a red light. My car came to a stop in the middle of the intersection. I apparently thought backing up was the right move to make. I threw the car into reverse and stepped on the gas. I felt an unexpected thud. My choice to back out of the intersection resulted in running into the car behind me. Within a few seconds, the car's driver pounded on my window. Being slow to react, I lowered my window. I could not tell you what was said if my life depended on it.

I do recall blowing a .12 alcohol level. In 1998 the legal blood alcohol level was at 0.10. Today the number is 0.08. I qualified for a ride to the Ottawa County Jail for an overnight stay to sober up. Handcuffs were tightened to my wrists as I was steered to the back seat of the police car. There I sat, meekly and calmly. This was mostly a result of the beer and pills. Between the booze and shock, I realized I had certainly screwed up this time.

The drive to the county jail in Grand Haven, Michigan, took thirty minutes. As I waited in an empty room. I became aware that correction officers do not move efficiently or fast. I think it has something to do with taxpayers' money. Where is the motivation to excel?

I had my fingerprints and photo taken. I remember trying to wipe the ink off, which only led to reapplying more. I was never shown the picture, nor do I ever want to see it. Some details are best left in the past. I was instructed to remove my belt, watch, and socks, along with any jewelry. I think I was given the chance to make one phone call which I chose to not make. I couldn't understand the recorded instructions being given.

I was then led to the holding cell where I remained until morning. The floor was covered with women, young, old, and middle aged—all haggard looking. Nobody looks good in jail. I found an area next to the stainless steel toilet. There was no pillow, and the blanket was cheap and thin. The lights continued to blaze overhead. I hoped sleep would come, but it did not. I was cold with no way to get comfortable. Just as I would settle down, another woman would be shoved through the door.

Morning finally came. While waiting to make my phone call, my belt, watch, and shoes were handed to me though a glass window. I dressed. My phone call was to James. Initially, he sounded relieved I was alive. He had frantically called the hospitals when I did not come back within an hour. As I left the building, I turned back and knocked repeatedly on the glass window where my belongings had been passed to me.

"You forgot to give me my keys and driver's license." The guard just stared at me and shook his head in disbelief. Has anyone ever looked at you with the "I can't believe this woman is so incredibly stupid look"? Yep, that's the one.

James studied me with great concentration as I climbed into the front passenger seat. By this time, he was thoroughly disgusted and angry with me. My actions were mortally wounding an already frail relationship. I just wanted a ride to my house and nothing more from him. Between the booze and the shock, my brain could not process any more. I think I had short circuited. It was a long, silent ride home.

I was free falling with two lead feet and had no idea of how to stop. A DUI at the age of forty seven…was I not supposed to be a responsible adult by now? I was too ashamed to admit to anyone my license had been revoked.

On November 17, I drove from my home in Hudsonville to the courthouse in Holland, Michigan, for my arraignment. I walked into the courthouse alone, trying to appear as nothing in my life had changed although everything in my day-to-day living was a lie. I lied to my parents, employer, and friends by saying nothing regarding the DUI. Continuing to drive without a license, I tried to stop drinking while driving, knowing another DUI would be devastating.

My case was the first to be addressed. Judge Jones asked me three times if I understood my plea of guilty. I responded, "Yes" each time. She seemed frustrated with my answer. The pressure of standing in the center of the courtroom became intense. I felt delusional at best. My final comment was, "I blew above the legal limit so I must be guilty." My driver's license was suspended for six months, and I was ordered to pay a fine and court costs.

As I left the courtroom, I felt smug. I had saved money by not hiring a lawyer. My goal was to resume driving without a license and no more drinking before or while driving.

Included in my sentence, I was to attend a four-hour DUI class on alcohol education. It was being held in a church west of Hudsonville. I made an attempt to drive to the church, and that is just what it was, an attempt. Of course, I drank before I left my home, became lost in a snowstorm, and arrived late. As I opened the door to enter the room, the instructor informed me in a loud voice, "The class has started. You will need to reschedule for next month." As I drove home, I blamed the weather, the instructor…I was only ten minutes late. Was it my fault the roads were not plowed? Oh well, another four weeks of driving illegally.

After two and a half months of driving without a license I requested a restricted license. I had read somewhere since I worked full time, I had a good chance of this request being granted.

I was ordered to appear in court on January 25 for my answer. I walked into the court room, late and alone. I quietly slid into the back row. Could it be my imagination or was Judge Jones staring at me? I cleared that thought out of my head. *I'm just being paranoid.* As I glanced around the court room, I noticed I was the only individual sitting alone. Everyone else was lawyered up.

Unlike my arraignment when I felt self-confident, this time my mouth was dry and the knot in my stomach was huge. My life was becoming more complicated. I felt on edge. From what I could perceive, Judge Jones denied every motion proposed by the lawyers. I had a bad feeling as I walked up to the center of the room for my turn before the bench.

"How did you get here today, Gail?"

What does this have to do with my restricted license proposal? I opened my mouth and the lies came pouring out. "My sister drove me."

"Where is she now?"

"She is shopping." *OMG another lie.*

"Well, when your sister drives here to pick you up, I would like to speak with both of you."

"Okay." I stammered and quickly left the room.

I walked to my car and sank into the driver's seat.

Now what? My response was simple. I purchased a six-pack of beer and elevated myself into a state of drunkenness while sitting in the parking lot of a convenience store. I then drove home, sat down, and conceded I was ready to attempt the unthinkable.

I would call Judge Jones while drunk, and under the influence of Ativan, which helped me feel self-confident, and Vicodin, which allowed me to escape my physical pain.

I couldn't believe I was being put through to the judge. She had very few words to say to me. "Gail, why don't you just admit you have been driving without your license?"

I had no response. All I could do was to agree to appear again in court on February 2 and admit to violating my probation. For that offense, I was given a three-day jail sentence.

For some reason they kept me in the Holland City Jail for my three-day sentence. I remember walking past two jails cells. The first was empty, and the second housed a lawbreaker/crook who had passed out on the floor. *I don't belong here.* I just have to wake up from this awful nightmare.

The next cell was for me. The area was approximately fourteen by twelve feet. There were no windows. Against the far wall was a cold, raised slab the size of a small twin bed—no mattress and no pillow, only a pea green, wool, frayed blanket. Placed on the right was a grimy, metal sink. The one object that stood out in my mind to this day was "the throne." *Why would one place that cold, steel object in the center of the room? What, no privacy?* In addition, where was the toilet paper? Nothing to read? The guard walked me in and handed me the blanket. I sat on the "bed," watched the cell door close with a grinding, reverberating sound. My sentence had begun.

Sitting in a county jail cell, I was nauseated, and every bone in my body ached. Add to this, the diarrhea had begun as a result of my body beginning to withdraw from the medications. I loved taking the Ativan especially. To summarize how it made me feel, "I felt as though a wave of relaxation washed over me." You take that drug away suddenly, cold turkey, and the feeling is indescribable...headache for three days straight, anxiety, and restlessness. I couldn't keep my legs from moving and sweating. I kept having nausea, vomiting, and diarrhea, lasting three days. The constant diarrhea left no break in the smell. Finally, yet importantly, my menstrual cycle commenced.

I have never felt more alone, sitting on the cold, metal toilet in the middle of my cell. I do not know who was more embarrassed, the male guard or myself when I asked for some tampons. He came back with one. I said I needed more than one. He made it clear I would be given one at a time. My response: "Do you think I'll attempt to hang myself by knotting them together?"

The overhead lights were on twenty-four/seven. Without my watch or a window to the outside world, I had no idea of the time. My attempts to sleep were overtaken by dreadful, horrible night-mares. One that occurred repeatedly was the feeling of drowning. I frantically tried to swim to the surface, but never was able. I would wake up gasping to breathe. No matter how I tried to wake up, I could not. I bit my lips as the diarrhea continued. My bottom lip was raw; I had a habit of biting my bottom lip when I was worried or anx-ious. I asked for some chap stick. I knew the answer to that request, "We do not stock that item."

As I exited the jail cell at midnight, I caught a glimpse of my mom and hung my head in shame. "I'm sorry, Mom." That's all I could say.

Chapter Two

MEMORIES OF MY MOTHER'S BEAUTY, her gentle laughter, and comforting touch, are always with me. I could, however, become so annoyed with her. For many years, she told me I was an alcoholic. I wonder how she could have known this. Was it so obvious?

I still find it surprising when I see alcohol being served in my hometown of Hudsonville, Michigan. As long as I lived there, one had to drive out of town to purchase alcohol.

My earliest memories are not infused with alcohol. My mother's father was an alcoholic, so there was very little drinking in my family when I was growing up. My family's history of not drinking was very different from many of the people I was in treatment with. Many were introduced to alcohol at a very young age, and alcohol was a steady theme throughout their childhood. I am unable to establish the reign or source of my drinking based on my home environment.

I have always felt insecure, both afraid and cautious, always wanting to do the "right thing." One example was at age five, in kindergarten, we would sit on a bench at the back of the room for story time. I had to go to the bathroom but was too afraid to tell my teacher. I started to cry. When my teacher asked me why I was crying I didn't answer. My best friend, Bonnie, raised her hand and said I had to use the bathroom but was afraid to ask. My teacher walked me to the small restroom, which was off from our classroom and not in the hall. I then proceeded to not come out. I must have been too scared. What a great memory from my first school year.

Maybe a better word to best describe my feelings would be anxious. Later in my life when I would have a drink, everything seemed softer. Life was more doable, but inside I was still a panicked five-year-old.

Bonnie was my best friend. We lived next door to each other growing up. I remember I wanted to be part of her family so bad. Bonnie had five siblings but I was always welcome to spend time at their house.

My dad had difficulty expressing his feelings, as did his father. We Dutch are naturally good at identifying and managing our emotions. My dad very seldom said, "I love you." However, he was the best father he knew how to be. I learned most of my compassion from my mother.

My brother, younger sister, and I attended a Christian School. There was always the annual disagreement over school selection in August because Christian school was expensive. My mom paid nearly the entire amount by doing housework in Grand Rapids. My dad would say public school was where we should be. I can remember I told them I didn't care where I went to school but to please just stop fighting.

In thinking back, I saw nothing in my childhood to suggest my history of becoming an alcoholic. I was not a latchkey kid. My mother was always home when I came home from school. I had chores to do around the house. My allowance was twenty-five cents a week for as long as I can remember.

We lived in a small, sheltered community, where no one had much privacy. On Sundays, church began at nine o'clock, followed by Sunday school, and evening church at seven o'clock. I'm grateful to have been rooted in church, as my faith in my "Higher Power "is a huge factor toward my sobriety today. However, as I grew older, I found myself thinking about rules I was told not to think about. At times breaking these rules consumed my thoughts as I wanted to be "normal." Normal at that time of my life would have included going to the movies, dancing, and riding my bike on Sundays.

Not watching TV on Sundays concluded around nine o'clock, since this was the time "Bonanza" aired, followed by "What's My Line." These were two of my father's favorite TV shows which he never missed.

Thankfully, the "no bike riding on Sunday rule" ended when Mom watched a local minister and his family riding their bikes past our house on a Sunday afternoon.

This brings us to the "no movie rule." My first movie was *The Sound of Music*. I don't remember what I told my mother my plans were for the evening. I recall sitting in this beautiful elegant movie theater with velvet curtains reaching to the ceiling. As the movie began, however, I had this sick feeling in the pit of my stomach. As I glanced up, I just knew the roof would somehow collapse, burying my body in the rubble. I pictured my mother wailing, asking, "Why would Gail do this?"

Next, the "No swimming on Sunday rules"—I dated a boy of the Catholic faith. This was definitely a "no no," especially with my father. Around noon one Sunday, we were eating lunch when the phone rang. It was John (the Catholic) asking if I wanted to go swimming with his family at a local country club.

"No," I mumbled.

"We will have a nice time. Are you sure you can't go?"

"I can't swim on Sunday," I explained.

"Can you swim on other days?"

"Yes, I stammered."

"I don't understand. If you can swim during the week, why are you unable to swim on Sunday?"

I told him I would not be going and would talk with him the next day. He really had no idea what I was talking about.

As far as alcohol consumption, there would be the occasional glass of Mogen David wine enjoyed by my parents on New Year's Eve. The bottle was then shoved back into the cupboard above the refrigerator. There it would remain for one year, waiting to be enjoyed once again on the holiday.

So ended the ceremony…occasionally, my dad would have one beer after work on a hot summer day. Add to the fact that Hudsonville was the last city in the county to be granted a liquor license, one could not just "run to the corner store" for more beer.

Both of my parents grew up during the Great Depression. My father grew up on a small dairy farm in Blendon Township. The village consisted of a church, gas station, grain mill, and country store. I remember Dad stating the family was not allowed to drink any milk since it was their livelihood. In fact, Dad was ahead of his time when it came to "using less than." We lived in the suburbs, no city water or sewer.

"Don't flush the toilet" was a familiar cry in our home. In fact, when I moved out into an apartment with friends, my habit of not flushing after every use became a problem. I was threatened with cleaning the toilets daily if something did not change.

"What about the septic tank?" I inquired?

"We live in the city." Okay then.

Our thermostat was forever set on low. Mom was always cold in the house, especially in the winter.

"Put some clothes on!" was another familiar shout.

One of the few opportunities Mom had to be warm was in the car. Dad would shove the heater into high gear. The heat in the car was "free of charge." By the time we would arrive at our destination, we would all be begging, "Turn it down."

One fact we could always count on was being the first car to arrive at church on Sunday morning. However, when my brother and I would start to get out of the car, Dad would say, "Not yet, we don't want to be the first people in church."

We always sat in the same seat every Sunday. "Fifth seat from the back on the right hand side," Dad would tell the usher.

My mom had a fear of sitting under the hanging lights at church, although there was never an incidence of one letting loose or falling on someone. And so, the Sunday regulations continued.

Dad was blue collar, a Democrat, and a Teamster. He was a truck driver for a local trucking firm that transported homegrown fruits and vegetables and was pro Jimmy Hoffa, who was president of the International Brotherhood of Teamsters, an American labor union. West Michigan had long been predominantly Republican; however, Dad was one of the few Democrats in Hudsonville. My mom was a Republican.

When Presidential Election Day came, the same scenario would unfold. Dad would walk into the house after a long work day. "Did you vote, Tim?"

If his answer was, "Yes," Mom would put her coat on and drive to the polls to cancel out his vote.

One more classic example of my childhood involved eating at Russ', a family-owned restaurant in Holland, Michigan. Every Saturday night, Dad would pull into the "drive in" section. My brother and I would always order a hamburger, French fries, and chocolate milk. We would sit on our knees, face the back window, and enjoy our meal. My sister is six years younger than me. As a child, she would order a cream chicken sandwich. When I would ask to have a chicken sandwich, I was told, "No." When I asked why my sister was allowed to eat chicken, I was told I liked hamburgers and she did not. *What?!*

Chapter Three

I WAS PROBABLY TWELVE before I realized a car could turn around and make unscheduled stops when going somewhere. Every year, the family vacation would consist of driving from Hudsonville "up north" to the bridge that connected the Lower Peninsula with the Upper Peninsula. Actually, we began taking this annual trip before the bridge was constructed.

I remember as early as 1957, when we often took the ferry to the Upper Peninsula. My only memory was my brother sitting on a container labeled, "adult life preservers."

When my brother asked where the children's life jackets were, my dad responded they didn't care about children. My poor brother never left his seat. My dad had a unique sense of humor.

My mom loved to stop at every gift shop on the way, but my Dad would say, "We are past the store, and we are not turning around."

This was before the four-lane highways. My dad would put forth all his effort in passing cars and trucks that were slow-moving. It would not be too long, and my mom would announce she had to use a bathroom. He would pull into a gas station, only to watch every vehicle he had overtaken drive by.

Our vacations always included my mother bringing all the food, sheets, towels, and washcloths. We would stay in cabins. I never realized how much work this involved until I was older. My dad would pull up to the office, Mom would get the key, and she would check out a cabin. If there was any musty smell or dirt, we would drive on to the next place.

We once vacationed at Niagara Falls, and it was different from our other trips. Our vehicle was basically too old to travel that distance so my dad borrowed my uncle's car for the trip. It was a white, 1958 Chevrolet. My parents decided we would stay in an actual hotel and eat out. I was so excited.

The night before we were to leave, there was a storm. A large tree in the back yard had fallen onto the garage. There was no structural damage, but it had to be cut up and transported away. That morning Dad saw the garage and made the decision we were not able to go. I am not sure what my mom said to Dad in their bedroom; however, he got up, packed the car, and we were off.

One more incredible event occurred. We were leaving Ontario when we saw a billboard asking if we took the tour and walked behind the falls. So the car turned around, and we went on the tour. I'm sure we must have stopped at several gift shops for Mom.

My mom loved shopping. I think I was eight when I remember Mom and I had been shopping most of the afternoon. We looked for a dress and finally found one that fit me. You can imagine how excited I was. We could go home!

I noticed Mom getting ready to go into another store. "Oh no! Why are you going to another store?" I cried.

Mother answered, "We might find one we like better."

Mom, my sister, and I would often travel. Mom would always have the items delivered after she arrived home. She did housework and had her "own money," but no sense in having my dad know everything.

In 2010 Mother passed. I am so thankful I stopped using drugs while Mom was alive. She never gave up on me.

I'm not sure why many of these memories are lodged in mind. When I conversed with my brother, he often responded, "I don't recall any of that."

In short, my younger years were typical. I grew up knowing my parents would always be at home when I got there or one call away. I cannot place anything in those early years that pointed toward addiction. My parents' occasional drink gave no clues to my adult alcoholism.

As mentioned earlier, my mother's father was an alcoholic, and she talked very little about her childhood. My mother despised drinking.

In order for me to stay sober, I have to combine Alcoholics Anonymous (AA) meetings and not have that first drink. Grandfather went to one AA meeting and never drank again. I believe if he had embraced AA, he would have received much needed support and understanding. He did the best he could do in his situation. Just think of the help he could have been to other alcoholics in the same situation he had experienced. He would have realized we are not bad people, but people with a bad disease. After all, technically he was "one of us."

My first job was actually when I was nine years of age. My brother and I "worked in the muck" topping onions. I was so excited! I remember waking Mom up early even though we rode our bikes. Topping onions involved pulling them out of the ground. When we had a hand full, we cut the onions from the stalk, and they would drop into the crate. It was very easy to cut your hands, and the juice from the onions would really bite. We were paid ten cents a crate.

There were a lot of us kids, and most of the time we had fun. Kool-Aid fights were popular. Only thing, if you wasted all your Kool-Aid, you had nothing to drink. Besides, Kool-Aid got real sticky when it dried.

As time went on, I eventually moved up to weeding flowers. I liked this more since there was no chance of injuring myself. At the top of my career I was able to "top" a hundred crates, totaling ten dollars a day! By the end of the season around the third week in August, I was sunburned, tired, and sore.

The man I worked for, as he paid us, said, "Now don't spend this all your money at the Hudsonville Fair." Sad to say that most of my money was spent there every year.

I also babysat for my neighbor's kids who lived across the street. My neighbor owned a local restaurant where I worked when I turned fifteen. Her children, were quite a handful. Oftentimes, they waited until the last minute to tell me they had to use the bathroom. I would take them to Hughes Park to play, and suddenly they would inform me the bathroom was needed. I would tell them to start running for home. However, when they stopped running, I knew it was too late. I guess you could say this was part of my on-the-job training to be a nurse!

When eleven years old in sixth grade, all of us girls had to watch a movie—the teachers said it was about "nursing." The boys already knew what the film was about before the girls did. It turns out the film broached the topic of crossing over to puberty.

Around the same time, I came home from school one day, and my mom insisted she needed to talk with me. She proceeded to discuss the same topic. I must have been shocked. She said, "Gail at least close your mouth."

Shortly afterwards, while outdoors playing street games with my neighbors, one of the boys informed me of the process for making a baby. I became physically sick and went home. I had planned on staying overnight at Bonnie's house but was too sick from his description.

Many years later I recognized him at a party. I could not restrain myself and asked if he remembered explaining sex to me. He did not and could not believe he had said those things.

As a seventh grader in 1963, I vividly remember when President John F. Kennedy was assassinated. We had a substitute teacher. Someone knocked on our classroom door and told our teacher the news. She came back into the room crying. When she shared what happened, some classmates laughed, not realizing it was true. She responded with shouting, "Did you hear what I said? The president has been shot!" We were dismissed.

About this time, the teachers expressed concern about my spelling. I took the "Iowa Basic Skills Test," which compared Hudsonville Schools with other schools across the county. My teacher called each of us to her desk, one by one, to review our results. When it came my turn, she said, "Let's talk about spelling. See this line on the graph? This is the national average, and this is you!" With that, she followed my line almost off the bottom of the paper. Her words of encouragement were: "Whatever you do, never become a secretary."

When I turned fifteen, I started to work at a local restaurant. On my first day at work, my mom took me in, and I remember sitting in the car and crying. Though I had a rough start, I worked there until after high school graduation. I worked with my good friend, Sally, who later went through nurses' training with me.

Chapter Four

AFTER ENROLLING into Pine Rest School of Nursing, one of our first assignments was to share why we chose nursing school. Many stated their mothers and grandmother were nurses. Several colleagues disclosed becoming a nurse had been a lifelong goal. My friend, Sally, and I made our decision based on being bored with working in the coffee shop and thought we would give nursing a try.

"I know what we can do! We can become nurses," I proposed.

It was settled. Our choice was health care vs. waitressing. We came to this decision within fifteen minutes. The teacher did not inquire as to any other facts.

Another perk of becoming a nurse turned out to be a big one.

We stayed on campus in Cutlerville, a suburb of Grand Rapids, and went home on weekends. In addition to our weekend trips, I enjoyed riding in a friend's pickup truck during the week, all the while drinking cheap wine and throwing empty bottles at road signs. This repeated itself every Wednesday. He was a bachelor who dined at the coffee shop daily, sometimes twice a day. You see, he had a massive crush on Sally, although feelings were not mutual. I still remember him pulling up to the dorm and honking his horn. This was our signal to jump into the truck. At the end of the evening, he would drive up to the door. This was my queue to jump out of the cab, which left Sally sitting next to him on the front seat. He would then stretch his right arm and put it around her. This was the farthest advance he ever made. Every Wednesday I would drink so much, I can still feel the entire room spinning as I crawled into bed. Someone suggested putting one foot on the floor would help, but I never found this true.

Sally was always trying to lose weight and found a doctor who would prescribe Dexedrine diet pills, also called amphetamines. I recall opening up some of her capsules and putting the powder in a container for myself. I only did this for a short time until Sally said the pills didn't help her anymore. I was afraid she would soon realize the capsules were not completely filled.

After graduation, I worked at Pine Rest, a psychiatric hospital, for several years. I found that performing a second shift gave me a better window to drink. For example, working three to eleven o'clock gave me time to drink after work with a group of friends. I would get to bed late but sleep in and repeated this routine several nights of the week. One night, while out, a coworker gave me some marijuana to try. I felt paranoid, so much so I did not finish the joint. I preferred to drink cheap wine during that time and later settled on beer as my drink of choice…Bud light or if someone else was buying, Heineken.

When I was younger, my mother suffered from postpartum depression after my sister's birth. At that time, electroshock therapy served as the primary treatment method, which was available at Pine Rest where Mom was treated. I remember visiting her and seeing her cry while sitting on the bed. While in nursing school, I observed a patient receiving this same treatment and passed out. It was just too difficult to watch. To this day, I don't know if this treatment helped. I can't remember asking my mom what it felt like or if her depression was lessened.

I turned twenty-one while in school. Several of us would get together after work and grab a pitcher of beer. I remember covering my glass with my hand and saying, "No thanks, I have had enough." My drinking did not involve rules. So, when did I stop wanting a drink and start needing a drink?

For many years I was happy and content with "normal drinking." Normal to me was one drink or maybe two during a scheduled event. Drinking was not part of my upbringing. There was no hint of any upcoming addiction.

After working at Pine Rest for two years, I applied for a position at a dermatology office. Carrie, a nurse I went to school with, called and said there was an opening for an LPN. This job really appealed to me—the beauty of dermatology is that very few people die from eczema, psoriasis, warts, and acne, although many of the conditions never go entirely away. Occasionally, we would see a melanoma, and they would be referred to a surgeon or oncologist. I worked there for five years and loved that job.

During this time, I married Harold and became pregnant. Abby was born in 1978, and Kristin was born in 1979.

Harold was someone who became less responsible as more responsibility came into our lives. He was hired at the railroad. The pay was good, although every six months, he would get laid off for at least four months. He enjoyed not working, but every other man I knew worked—my father, brother, etc. During the time he was off, I worked weekends at the dermatology office and nights at the Hudsonville Christian Nursing Home. I would come home at seven o'clock in the morning, tired after working all night, and would find the house a total disaster. He did not do the dishes nor pick up the place after the girls went to bed. Often, he would be asleep on the couch, and Abby and Kristin would be running about. I finally told him to leave. He lived with his parents and never came back into the house…not because he did not want to. I said, "No," and later filed for divorce.

I remember going to a marriage counselor during this time. He suggested I ask Harold to do some "fix it" jobs around the house. For example, replace a burned-out light bulb in the garage. My response: "Why should I ask him to do that? He never changed a light bulb as long as we were married. That just doesn't make sense."

That was my last counseling session.

Harold's foster parent continued to be a part of our lives. They took their family to Disney World, and Abby, Kristin, and I were included, as well as at family gatherings, holidays, celebrating birthdays, etc. The girls enjoyed swimming in their pool during summers. They also helped out financially. I still call "Mother T" often. At age ninety-four, she sounds like she did forty years ago…a very giving person, and I am so glad we have kept in touch over the years.

I drank very little in my twenties and thirties. I worked full-time raising Abby and Kristin as a single mom. Kristin, my youngest daughter, was born with a condition called Neurofibromatosis (NF). In some cases, tumors can grow along nerves. I took her to my previous employer, the dermatologist. She was born with several small light tan areas, called Café' au lait spots, on her hand and stomach area. Although they do not occur frequently, complications can develop. And yes, this was Kristin's case. No one in our family history has had this condition. Fifty percent of the cases are genetic, and fifty percent are spontaneous mutations.

When Kristin was three, she developed a tumor in her optic nerve. I noticed her left eye looked more down and slightly protruded. We were referred to Ann Arbor and then to Toronto Hospital for Sick Children. What a terrible name! Of course, children in a hospital are sick. The floor where Kristin was admitted provided care for children with head tumors. It was the most depressing place I had ever seen. They offered no hope for her.

I remember the doctor asked why we were there. Naturally, we were there for Kristin to receive treatment for her condition.

"Take her home and enjoy whatever time she has left." That was the doctor's advice.

I worked nights at the nursing home. My sister would stay over-night with the girls. During this time in my life, I never thought of drinking. My young daughters needed their mother and not a drunk mother. I'll never forget the events that resulted in Kristin's treatment. One of the dermatology doctors came in at midnight to see a resident. I worked eleven o'clock in the evening to seven o'clock in the morning. He had never made a "house call" at this time before. He asked me how I was doing. I just broke down and cried. He asked if he could call me the next day with some ideas. Of course, I said, "Yes."

He had recently referred a patient to Will's Eye Hospital in Phil-adelphia, Pennsylvania. Within a week, Kristin had an appointment. Although they couldn't treat her, they referred her to Children's Hos-pital of Philadelphia (CHOP). We stayed at the first Ronald McDon-ald House while in Philadelphia. They suggested a clinical trial with chemotherapy to destroy the tumor behind her eye. Chemotherapy targets cells that grow and divide quickly, as cancer cells do. Even though NF cells are not cancerous, in Kristin's case, the cells were dividing at an abnormally rapid rate. She had already lost most of her vision in her left eye. In looking back at her young age of three, I had attributed her cautious walking to being naturally slow-moving. I felt sad that we had lost valuable time in her treatment.

We were thrilled with the treatment plan and headed home. The trial would be coordinated through a pediatric hematologist in Ann Arbor and local hematologist in Grand Rapids. She was on weekly chemotherapy in the Grand Rapids office, and one week a month in Ann Arbor for two years.

Our doctor in Ann Arbor was a gift from God. Our first consult visit was scheduled, and the appointment was with another doctor. I was told the doctor we were referred to was unable to take any new patients. I thought for a moment and explained to them he was the doctor we had been referred to by CHOP, and he was the doctor I wanted for Kristin. As Kristin's treatment continued, I told him several times I often accepted changes, but standing my ground was the best choice I could have made. He was such an excellent doctor and such a special person. If he said he would return my call or commit to doing something else, I knew he would follow through.

At that time in my life, I believe I did not have time to drink. I worked three jobs. Thank the Lord for my family! My sister would stay nights, while I worked third shift at the nursing home. I eventually worked for the hematology office full time. The doctors said I was at the office so much I may as well work there.

That was my dream job for eighteen years. It was also the job I was fired from for was using drugs and alcohol. It is sad to say when I was fired, I really realized I needed to stop. Apparently, losing my job meant more to me than the respect of my family and friends.

I was fired in 1999. By this time, I was calling in my own prescriptions to local pharmacies. I was so high when I went to pick up a prescription for pain medications that I had called in for myself...I did not remember I had picked it up earlier in the afternoon. After the pharmacist told me I had picked it up, he called my office to speak with the doctor to let him know one of his patients was taking too much medication. When he gave the doctor the patient's name, he was shocked. "There must be some mistake. Gail is not my patient; she is my nurse!"

Chapter Five

THINGS WEREN'T ALWAYS crazy, though. For a while, my life finally seemed to be more regular. I worked at Hematology, Kristin and Abby were doing well. Once a month, Kristin, Abby, my mom, and I would drive to Ann Arbor, where we would stay for one week, while Kristin was an inpatient for her chemotherapy. Eventually she went into remission.

Several years later, I met Mike. We were so happy together. Both of our first marriages had been miserable. We married a year after we met. Mike was an engineer at General Motors. I believe he was the only man I dated that my dad could say nothing wrong about. (Dad only bought GM cars!)

Mike and I usually enjoyed a couple beers when eating out, but I never drank to get drunk. Abby and Kristin got along with Mike, too. Our lives were perfect! It was a minor adjustment for them since they were used to having me all to themselves.

It wasn't too long after we were married, I noticed Mike seemed to be short of breath. He would blow it off when I brought it up. We went to his primary care physician, who referred Mike to a pulmonary doctor. After a lung biopsy, Mike was diagnosed with pulmonary fibrosis. I can still hear the pulmonary doctor explain, "Pulmonary fibrosis usually smolders along for years with no debilitating symptoms. He will lead a normal life with medication." Unfortunately, that was not the case for Mike. His disease progressed quickly.

He was the type of person who always had to be doing something. After his diagnosis, I did everything in my power to prevent him from overdoing it. He left to go to work before me. If he would tell me there was a task he wanted to do when he came home, I would get out of bed after he left and do whatever he had planned. I would leave him a note saying I couldn't sleep, so I would do the chore he had planned on tackling and he could rest.

One day, we had returned home from an appointment with his pulmonary doctor. I remember standing in the kitchen. We held each other, both crying. I remember him saying, "I don't want to die."

I also remember watching a movie on TV. One of the scenes involved being filmed underwater. He couldn't watch it. He felt like he was already underwater, drowning.

Mike was in and out of the hospital several times. He was on a ventilator in the intensive care unit (ICU), where one of the nurses waited to talk with us. His daughter, was with me. We sat in a small room,

The nurse said, "This may be Mike's last admittance."

At first, I did not realize what he was talking about. "Was the insurance running out?" I asked.

The nurse quietly said he would not make it home again.

That was the night he coded and passed. This was ten days short of our being married a year. The nurse told me he was no longer suffering. He was in a place where there is no pain. That thought seemed to comfort me. However, by the time I drove home, I just wanted him back with me.

I seriously thought of pulling my car in front of a train. I knew I could never do that. My daughters needed me. It was around this time I started taking samples of pain medications and anti-anxiety medicine from the office stock—not because I was in pain, but strictly for the way, I felt when taking them. The pain medications would hype me up, and the Ativan (anti-anxiety) would help me sleep.

During 1991, the year Mike was sick, I did not take care of myself. Having two daughters, age twelve and thirteen, Mike's illness, and working seemed to leave little time for me.

Six months after he passed away, I began to have stomach issues. I lost weight, had no appetite, and just did not feel well at all. In looking back, I had these symptoms for quite some time. Nurses are notorious for not caring for themselves. There were gastrointestinal (GI) doctors in the medical building I worked in, so I finally scheduled an appointment. After being scoped, I apparently had an ulcer I had ignored for many months. Scar tissue had formed where my stomach emptied into my small intestine. My stomach would no longer empty. That day, I was admitted to a local hospital in Grand Rapids where I had two surgeries, which were unsuccessful over the next twelve weeks.

I couldn't believe this was happening to me. I had never been sick and had never been hospitalized. I did not eat for three months—the entire time I was an inpatient. I also celebrated my fortieth birthday in the hospital. A nasogastric tube was placed up my nose into my stomach. Suction was then applied to continuously remove stomach contents and deposit them into a container on the wall behind my bed. This is one of the most painful procedures I have ever had. I developed ulcers up and down my throat. Several times it had to be changed, and this was in place for four months. My nourishment came from Total Parenteral Nutrition (TPN) fed through a central line, which is a catheter placed in a large vein near the heart. More nourishment came from a feeding tube placed into my small intestine.

During this time, I felt I was going crazy from this situation. I was so restless I couldn't read the cards I received. I only read who they were from. Thank the Lord for my family. They were always doing whatever they could to help. At this time I was given Ativan for my anxiety and pain medication for pain after the two surgeries. I know they were concerned about the medications since both were addictive drugs. I gradually took less and less.

I only was allowed to have some ice chips during these months. Whatever I swallowed was removed out of my stomach into a container on the wall. After watching TV, commercial after commercial of food and drink, I was able to talk a friend into bringing me a Schweppes ginger ale. My plan was to sip it slowly. Unfortunately, I lost control and drank the entire can at once. You can imagine how surprised the nurse was when she came into the room. The whole can of liquid was now in the container on the wall. I promised I would never do that again.

Finally, I talked my doctors into letting me go home with my machines and pumps. My family gave so much of themselves to help Abby, Kristin, and me during this time. My mom did not want me to come home, though, because she was afraid I would not be able to handle the feeding machines and dressing changes. A visiting nurse was scheduled for several visits, but after one I told her I was okay. I "unhooked" myself once a day and walked half a mile every day. Abby helped me mix my IV fluids.

I decided to have my last surgery in Ann Arbor. After being home for four weeks, I had healed enough for them to remove ninety percent of my stomach. During my stay, several tornadoes were spotted near the hospital. I had just had surgery and had not been out of bed when a tornado warning sounded. I was lifted out of bed, thrown in a chair, and dragged into the hallway. I remember thinking, *please, don't let me be blown away after all I've gone through.*

My first meal in four months included a large portion of beef stroganoff. Apparently, portions had not been discussed with the dietary department. As I delved into the meal, I suddenly did not feel well. I rang for the nurse. My doctor told me to start walking and not to stop until he told me to. A scan was ordered, and thankfully none of the sutures had separated. My new portion was a quarter slice of bread.

Today I still have to work at maintaining my weight. My portions are not huge, but I feel good. I have learned when and what I should eat. I was off work for six months and required physical therapy since I had been in bed for four months. I seemed to be on track.

At this point, I should have been back to my everyday family/work responsibilities without medication. Instead, I found myself taking samples from my office. Taking pain medications with alcohol enhanced my energy even more. Alcohol would take the "edge off." I felt focused and creative. The samples I took—cough medicine with codeine, pain pills, Benzodiazepines such as Xanax and Valium, were there for patients who did not have insurance.

If one of the doctors commented, "I thought we had samples of pain meds and sleeping pills," I would shrug my shoulders and appear to be too busy to respond. It wasn't long when taking samples was not satisfying my need to use. I needed plan B. I decided to call in my own prescriptions.

The first call was to my local pharmacy (There was only one in Hudsonville). I phoned them in under my name as the patient, using my insurance card to pay. Bad choice! It wasn't very long before the pharmacy and insurance picked up that I was calling for myself. After all, the pharmacist recognized my voice and put two and two together. I still remember the sick feeling in my gut when the pharmacist asked to speak with my employer.

"I would like to speak with you, Gail, before you go home," my boss said.

At the end of the day, he confronted me in his office. He said the pharmacist had called out of concern for me. (Really? Pharmacists loved making trouble for people. I wasn't hurting anyone.)

He asked if I needed help stopping. Of course, I said, "Absolutely not. I can stop on my own." He had done some investigating and found a long-term inpatient treatment program in Grand Rapids. I agreed (like I had a choice) to meet with the addictionologist. He asked me if any of my family were alcoholics. My answer: "No, not that I am aware of." I knew where this conversation was going. If I said, "Yes," he would use this in his favor. This would increase the odds of me being an alcoholic. His recommendation was that I be admitted into his four-month inpatient treatment program. *He is after my insurance money.*

Before I left, I agreed to go to a Caduceus Meeting that evening, which consisted of all health-care professionals ranging from medical doctors, pharmacists, and dentists, to nurses and veterinarians. The caduceus is a Greek medical symbol. This group was terribly intimidating…the only way I made it through the hour and a half meeting was by taking several Ativan. I sat and listened to forty health-care professionals "check-in."

The check-in went as follows: "Hello. I am Joe Blow, an alcoholic addicted doctor from Grand Rapids." As everyone checked in, one would ask for time to talk during the hour and a half. Finally, I was the last person to check in. I followed the format and said I had nothing to talk about. One of the doctors asked me if I thought I was an alcoholic, to which I answered, "Yes." I would have said anything to get out of that room. Little did I know, eight years from that day, in 1999, I would resurface in that very room.

The following day I told my employer I decided to go to Pine Rest for outpatient treatment. Two reasons for my choice were it was covered by my insurance, and it was a Christian hospital—what a joke. I never took that treatment seriously. I said what they wanted to hear.

Chapter Six

I WAS ABLE to get my drinking and using drugs somewhat under control. I did not call any prescriptions in for a long time. That meeting with the health-care professionals scared me enough to be more cautious. Many of the people I was in treatment with later would talk about their need to not hang around with their "drinking friends" when they stopped drinking. As it turns out, I drank the most of any of my friends.

My sister and I always had a good time going out bar hopping. One comment she would make at the end of the night was she was "beered out." What?!

We often went on trips together, too. Key West, Florida, was a favorite destination. We would travel light, mainly with just shorts and a T-shirt, drinking our way across the island. I actually stopped using any pills.

In 1993, we spent a short four-day weekend in St. Louis, Missouri. After unpacking, we met in the bar around five o'clock in the afternoon. My sister was talking with two cute guys, who invited us to attend the Junior Achievement. International Convention.

As we were on the shuttle bus, we were informed a picture ID with our name and state was a requirement to enter the convention. Newt Gingrich was the keynote speaker, and people speculated he would be running for president the next election year. Naturally, we wanted to hear him speak. We waited in the lobby while the two guys found two girls, they believed resembled us. We were able to use their identification badges and walked through security without a problem. Newt had just entered the center aisle and made his way to the stage.

Within a few minutes, I waited in the beer line. A tall, stocky young man tapped me on my shoulder. "Hi, Jane," he said. "Are you having a good time?"

"Yes, Bob. How about you?" (I read his name tag.)

"I'm not sure who you are, but I know you are not Jane."

"Busted, can I buy you a beer or two?"

After returning the name tags to the rightful owners, We spent the rest of the evening visiting people from the various states represented and ended the evening listening to Newt speak. We sat with representative from the great state of Hawaii. We couldn't have stuck out more if we tried.

The following day we toured the Budweiser brewery. I'm proud to say we both polished off two beers within the fifteen-minute time limit!

Every year, four of us nurses who had worked together would drive or take the train to Chicago for a weekend. Our first stop would be the Walgreens on Michigan Avenue, where we would purchase our alcohol for our stay. I was always the one who wanted "just one more drink." One of the women actually polished off a bottle of whisky in three days and two nights. Of course, her bottle was a recycled airline bottle approximately two inches tall. I remember being concerned about being with girlfriends my first year in recovery. I found out they were only drinking because I drank. We continued to enjoy our sober times together for many years.

Chapter Seven

MY DAUGHTER, Kristin, was in high school at this time. Her goal in life was to find every pill and can of beer in the house. I hid them all over the place. I feel so sad and ashamed for what I put her through. Every time she would leave the place to go out with friends, she would ask, "You're not going to drink tonight, are you, Mom?"

My answer was always, "No," and every night I went against my word. I would be so angry with her. I remember she went to our primary care physician for a cold. She told me she talked with the doctor about me. The doctor suggested she move out of our home to get away from me. I was shocked. I couldn't believe she said that about me. Plus, I couldn't believe he suggested she move away from her mother. I lived in such denial. Kristin should never have had to go through this. I had not been a mother to her for so long.

Kristin would check my car for beer every day when I came home from work. She could hear me crack open a beer can a mile away. In the winter, I would drop cans of beer in the shrubbery along the driveway. After she would go to bed, I would go out and dig in the snow to find them. As I look back at this time in my life,

I feel physically sick…so much time and effort spent, wasted.

When writing this, Kristin has passed away from an inoperative brain tumor. My only relief from this pain is she lived to see me sober for eighteen years. It took many years for her to trust me again. I had to earn that trust. There is a saying often mentioned at one of my favorite AA meeting groups, The Old Timers: "Show me, don't tell me." Hopefully, at some point, I showed her.

My addiction seemed to smolder along for several years. I dated James for a total of six years, beginning in 1993. He worked for one of the largest law firms in Grand Rapids.

We met at a restaurant in downtown Holland for a drink. Odd, I remember very little of the conversation that evening. I do remember he did not order a drink. He said he had a cold. (What does a cold have to do with not drinking?)

On the other hand, I had two beers and pre-medicated myself with Ativan, just to take the edge off. An alcoholic is unable to determine what a stressful situation is. We tend to treat every new situation as stressful. I compare this to health-care workers, who are taught to treat all blood contact as positive for HBV or HIV.

I think I felt inferior dating James. I felt "less than," which is a common trait of alcoholics. He was nine years older than me and financially very comfortable. We vacationed together several times.

My first cruise was with James. I believe we were gone for ten days. Being gone this length of time took excellent planning… not my wardrobe, but trying to get together enough pills to last the entire trip. By this time, I was calling in my own "scripts" again. I tried to stock up and pace myself. My use was still manageable. I divided my pills into neatly organized containers. As we introduced ourselves at the dining table. James told the waiter he would like several bottles placed on his tab. To my surprise, James and I were the only two at the table who drank. I believe drinking was against their religion (like that ever stopped me). An announcement was made after the first meal if anyone wanted their seating changed to feel free to notify your waiter.

Yes, I wanted my seating changed. *Seven days seated at a table with religious people who do not drink! OMG, what fun is that?!*

Of course, I did not want to admit this, so I was forced to squeeze in a beer here and there when James and I separated. I also always carried a map with me, not wanting to get lost. We had an enjoyable time although I always wanted to drink more than James did, and feel guilty for those thoughts.

Another vacation we took together was to Key West. We signed up for a sunset cruise. I figured we would sail just offshore, throw the anchor, and enjoy all the champagne we wanted. The further we sailed into the Gulf, the more seasick I became. People took turns steering the boat. When my turn came, I was in the bathroom vomiting. However, I grabbed a bottle of champagne as we docked since I had been too sick to drink on board.

On the flight home, we were not sitting together for some reason. He said he would try to trade seats to sit with me after takeoff. As we waited to take off, I heard him talking loudly and laughing with the female passenger sitting next to him. On the overhead announcement, they mentioned the airline offered two free round-trip tickets and $250 in cash. That's all I needed to hear. I stood up, reached overhead for my carry-on and started to walk off the plane. The last thing I heard was someone saying, "James, she's getting off the plane!" after which he said, "No, she would never do that." Yes, I did. Looking back on this part of my life is exhausting. When I combined pills and booze, my actions were unpredictable.

I would get out of work at five o'clock in the afternoon, open a beer, and drink while driving to his house in Holland. I would drink another one while taking a shower. We enjoyed a bottle of wine while cooking and enjoying dinner. On my drive home, I would stop at the same gas station and purchase a six-pack of beer and a bag of popcorn. I believe James was unaware of my drinking on the way to his house and on the drive home. He always asked that I give him a call when I arrived home. Most of the time, I would forget to call as I had passed out in bed. The next day he would ask me why I didn't call him. I would say I just felt too tired and apologize. Truth being, I had more than likely had a blackout and did not even remember the drive home.

On hot, summer days, I would often buy ice and a twelve-pack of beer on my lunch hour and put it in my trunk. Summer was my favorite time of year. With road construction, I usually slammed three "cold ones" on the way home due to the 45-mph speed limit.

Sometimes I would buy some cheese and crackers and veggies and dip for my own "Happy Hour." It was only by the grace of God I never caused an accident.

Once in the winter, I slid off the road as a car passed me. No one was hurt, and the driver called the police. Sitting in the back seat of the cop car, he asked me to do a breathalyzer, which I did.

"I could book you right now for a DUI." Instead, he drove me home to my condo. Of course, I promised to never drink and drive again. I'm sure this was a night I never gave James a call. In fact, I never remembered this situation until I was an inpatient at the long-term treatment center several years later.

During this time period, I attempted to see a therapist, who said a new treatment option consisted of only drinking two beers and only two whenever I was out and wanted a beer. You can only imagine my surprise when she told me this as her therapy. I named this "my control method." The only result I saw from this therapy was that I spent more money purchasing two, then going back for more. In looking back, I think this was her way of showing me that I was an alcoholic.

I tried eating healthy, but it was a no-brainer choice to drink or eat. Drinking won every time. I purchased a computer, hoping I would become addicted to my laptop vs. beer. I would often call my girlfriends late at night or early in the morning, of course, drinking the entire time. I tried to make notes of what we talked about, but was unable to read my own writing.

Since my "treatment" at Pine Rest, it was suggested I attend AA.

I remember my first AA meeting, called "The West Coast Club." The place was far from a club. My mom had driven me to the meeting since, at this time, I had lost my driver's license from my DUI.

I remember sitting in the car, not wanting to get out. I did not want to go to any meeting, but most of all, I was scared to get out. The meeting was in a large smoke-filled room. Approximately twenty people, mostly men, sat around an oblong table. I think there were only five women. From what I can recall, everyone drank coffee and smoked. As I looked around the table, I remember thinking, *I don't want to be here, I don't belong here. These drunks have stringy, greasy, gray hair.* Some of them even had teeth missing!

What was the worst, this was my first meeting. When the chairman asked if anyone was here for their very first meeting any time, any place, I raised my hand. (I later learned that many alcoholics do not raise their hand and admit to it being their first meeting. How odd that thought never occurred to me.) The rest of the hour-long meeting was directed at me. Every person told me how their life had been, what happened, and how their life was today. This was a very long one-hour meeting for me. Although the length was only sixty minutes, I could not get out of that room soon enough.

It is odd how certain moments or thoughts can remain in your mind. I remember seeing a note being passed from one person to another. My name was written on a folded piece of paper. One short line read, "You don't have to take the elevator all the way down." I glanced across the table and smiled at the middle-aged lady who wrote this note. I was smiling on the outside, but I could not believe these people. As if this one-hour meeting wasn't bad enough, these losers were actually talking about getting together for a picnic the coming weekend. (You see, I had not reached the basement of my elevator shaft, yet!)

One of my favorite therapy sessions was my last visit with another social worker in Zeeland, Michigan. She always offered me a cup of office coffee, which I gladly accepted. However, this morning I brought my own coffee to which I had added some Baileys Irish cream. It never entered my mind that my speech may have been somewhat altered or she might smell the aroma. When she suggested I attend a "great AA meeting Friday night at a local church," I laughed. "Friday night is my night." As I left, I agreed when she stated I did not need to make a return visit.

There was a body shop in Hudsonville where I would take my car when I scraped it, knocked the mirror off, backed up into a cement post in a parking lot, etc. I learned I could not submit any claims to my auto insurance for fear of my rates going up. And I certainly didn't want anyone to get the idea I might be drinking and driving! Therefore, I was forced to pay for my repairs with cash.

As I paid for, yet another repair job in Hudsonville, the owner stood back, arms folded, and said, "I believe we have replaced every part of this car twice." I knew it was time to get my repairs made out of town. You see, I had this crazy idea if I drove a car without dents and scratches, it must mean I was not an alcoholic.

When I look back at that time in my life, I find it amazing I was unaware of how unmanageable my life was becoming. For example, when I picked up my car from the body shop for replacing the driver's side rearview mirror, I knocked the mirror off as I pulled up to the drive-through window at the bank. On my way home, I decided to withdraw some cash. As I drove away, I again ran into the same pole, and the same mirror cracked off.

I had not even made it home. One definition of insanity is "doing the same thing over and over, but expecting different results."

I would get up in the morning to go to work and find a dent, scrape, or flat tire. This must have occurred on my drive home from somewhere in a blackout. A blackout is a classic symptom of an alcoholic. I remember my stay at the Betty Ford Center. A woman was there for twenty-eight days and then to prison with the charge of vehicular manslaughter. She was involved in an accident and was responsible for the death of a young child. That could have been me over and over. When I hear of a drunk driver going the wrong way on the expressway, I always feel like he or she more than likely does not remember what occurred.

It was around this time I finally talked with my primary care provider about my addiction. I did not mention my taking prescription drugs, only alcohol. I also took time off work but did not tell my employer the reason. There is a saying in AA: "Half-truths availed us nothing."

I excelled in half-truths, half-efforts, never fully committing. That is one reason it took me so long to stop using. My health-care provider admitted me to a five-day in-patient center for detox. Shortly after arriving, I began asking when I could go home. The doctor asked me why I wanted to go home. The correct answer was to drink and use. Some of my reasons were, "My job, my children, etc..."

There was one person there who was also a nurse, and he was there to "save his job." In truth, I related to everyone there. I was an alcoholic... after five days, I was formally discharged. So much for my first inpatient treatment.

I did not stop drinking.

In fact, my use of drugs continued to increase. I had a list of ten local pharmacies I would call. Keeping track of names, dates of birth, and addresses became a monumental task. A wave of fear always swept over me as I walked into the pharmacy and gave my fictitious name. If the pharmacist would walk to the phone, I knew he or she could be calling the police to tell them I was at their pharmacy. Sometimes I would leave without picking up the "script" just out of fear. I had heard stories of police waiting to arrest someone as they walked out of the store. This happened to another nurse I later met in treatment.

I remember my therapist asked me if I thought the pharmacist remembered me.

I said, "No."

Did I remember them?

"Yes"

Say no more. Point made.

The sick feeling of walking into a pharmacy continued for several years, even after I was clean. Eventually, this anxiety led to a natural high. What could be better than picking up a prescription at the same pharmacy that was legal? Yay!

Being addicted to drugs and alcohol is not "having a good time." Those days are gone forever. Alcoholics all suffer from the human condition of not knowing how to deal with life on life's terms. I can remember my first day in long-term treatment. I stood looking at the closed door thinking, "I don't think I can do this without alcohol or drugs."

After being "caught" by my employer when calling in pills, I was given a "Last Chance Agreement" with random urines. I did not go back to work at this time, but focused on my stay at the Betty Ford Center.

Chapter Eight

SEVERAL DAYS PASSED before I was able to rearrange my flight and my stay out to Palm Springs.

My sister and James had done somewhat of an intervention. My choices for treatment were Hazelton in Minnesota or the Betty Ford Center (BFC) in Palm Springs, California. This was in February of 1999. My selection was a no-brainer, Betty Ford Center in Palm Springs.

My boyfriend of six years at the time, James, agreed to drive me to the Grand Rapids International Airport. If he pointed out one more time, the importance of not drinking on this flight, I would have started screaming.

"Yes, I absolutely flushed all my pills down the toilet."

"Yes, James, I promise I will not drink." *Why can't he give me some credit? After all, tomorrow, I will be checking myself into BFC.*

As we touched down in Chicago. I barely had time to slam down one beer. My prescription drugs, Darvocet, Tylenol 3, and Ativan, were safely packed in my carry-on, along with a generous number of loose pills in my pockets. I made a quick pocket check. I was only in

Chicago for a short layover. At least I had enough sense not to drink down several cold ones in the airport. I didn't want to be one of those obnoxious drunks not allowed to board. As the plane leveled off, I washed down several more pills with my drink. I finally fell asleep, or to be more accurate, I passed out.

The next thing I knew, our plane had touched down in Los Angeles, and passengers were disembarking from the aircraft. I honestly have no recall of stumbling my way to the Northwest terminal. As I boarded for the short commuter flight to Palm Springs, I'm sure it was pretty obvious where my final destination would be—the BFC!

After finding my luggage, I flagged a taxi and crawled into the back seat. I had made reservations at one of the local hotels in Palm Springs which offered a discount rate to those "checking in" to the BFC. After taking care of the check-in process, I was now ready to move on to more urgent needs.

"Where can I buy some beer? "I asked the gentleman at the front desk.

"All stores have already closed," he replied.

Closed! There has to be a convenience store open. It was early in the night, eleven-thirty. After much whining, he said there was one store approximately a half mile down the road, but it was in a questionable area. Since I had no car or driver's license, I thanked him and headed to the exit. He caught up to me and said he had a couple beers in his refrigerator in the back room, and I was welcomed to have those. *Two? What good are two? We are talking about some last-call drinking...*

you know, the "I'm going into treatment for drugs and alcohol in the morning drinking."

The sad thing was I never thought of being a responsible person, having something nutritious to eat, taking a shower, and getting some rest after my cross-country air trip. But then sensible thinking had long since left me. As I opened the door to walk down the street, I heard the desk clerk utter, "Alright, get in my car, and I will drive you."

As I stood in front of the cooler, I remember thinking, "A six-pack or will I need twelve for the night?" To my surprise, a twelve-pack of my favorite was on sale. There was my answer; twelve it was. We road back to the hotel in silence. As I opened the car door, I remember his question, "Will you be alright?"

Alright! Wow, several years earlier, this evening would have been so far from my alright, but tonight I answered, "Yes, I will be just fine." I quietly thanked him as I pushed the car door closed.

As I threw my suitcase on the bed, I glanced around the room for the refrigerator. *Okay, I really just need some ice.* I placed at least seven cans in the bathroom sink. After several trips to the ice machine, I was able to sit back and relax. I set the alarm for seven o'clock. I was to call the BFC at eight o'clock in the morning. After the phone call, a driver would pick me up in the hotel lobby.

One of the requirements—rules before checking into the center—was absolutely no alcohol consumption for twenty-four to forty-eight hours. The reason was that if someone stopped cold turkey, they could possibly experience dangerous seizures. BFC is not located in a medical facility. The nearest one was the Eisenhower Medical Center several miles east of the clinic. Was I aware of this regulation? Yes, of course, I was. Why, then, was I drinking as I placed my 8:15 call in the morning? Because I am an alcoholic and the thought of not drinking never entered my mind.

As my call was transferred to the appropriate intake person, it must have been undeniable I had been drinking for some time.

"Gail, you know we cannot admit you if you have been drinking in the past twenty-four hours."

My response: "No worries, I have plenty of pills and beer to last me all weekend. I'll be just fine."

"We are sending a driver to pick you up at once. He will meet you in the lobby." So, my twenty-eight days stay began.

Chapter Nine

CHECKING INTO BFC drunk was quite an experience. My suitcase was taken from me.

I was told to pack everything I might need for the entire twenty-eight days since I would not be able to leave on my own or go to any nearby stores. I believe there was a maximum of twenty-four women inpatient at all times. I was not allowed to keep my curling iron, hair spray, or perfume. Later we found out a patient drank her entire bottle of perfume and died as a result. The mouthwash was to be alcohol-free only.

I wanted to stay in my room and sleep, but was allowed only an hour to rest. I was later told the admitting team was amazed I could get up every morning that first week. We would check in every morning at the medical clinic, where our blood pressure and pulse would be checked. They had an interesting method of who was next in line to be seen. The time to be seen was from seven to eight o'clock. One would walk into the waiting room and ask, "Who is last?" Whoever answered "I am" was the person you were behind in line.

Also, the first check-in was more thorough, more details were asked. A perfect example was when they asked how many pills and how much drinking did I do every day. Of course, I minimized the numbers. As I began to withdraw, my symptoms became more obvious as I was unable to sleep. Still, if I dozed off, the nightmares would be terrible. I would shower at least twice during the night because of severe pain in every muscle of my body. By the third day, my blood pressure and pulse became dangerously high. I remember the nurse saying, "Are you ready to be honest and tell me the correct number of drugs you were taking?"

At that point, I didn't care about any numbers. I just wanted my intense pain to go away. I was given a patch of some kind that they placed on my back and several other medications to ease the symptoms. In fact, I can remember sitting in the cafeteria after lunch. As others were leaving, I remained seated. I told them I would sit back a bit because I felt a little high and wanted to enjoy the feeling.

"We understand perfectly."

When I was first admitted, they drew blood work that showed my liver enzymes as elevated. I was really shocked. I think it was a reality check-proof…I really was an alcoholic, and I really should have cared about my numbers.

Quite honestly, though, I do not remember too much of the check-in process during which I was drunk, high, and in a blackout. As time went on, many people would say, "Hi Gail." It seemed they obviously knew who I was, but why did I not remember them? When I would ask how I was supposed to know them, responses ranged from "I picked you up at the hotel, or I took your picture when you were admitted, or I charged your credit card $12,000.00." Another growth spurt was watching my various black and blue marks gradually fade away. The color would go from blue to yellow to tan and gone! I never realized how often I bumped or scraped myself when I was drunk.

My generalized aches and pain gradually lessened as the month went on. However, my sleep did not improve. One of the doctors told me I would not have a night of normal sleep for ninety days. This was due to the Ativan medication I had taken every night just to fall asleep. Being at BFC for twenty-eight days did not stop me from ever using again, but I did learn I never wanted to withdraw from Ativan again. I never took that medication again.

There was another reason I did not fall asleep. I was in the habit of watching TV to fall asleep. Televisions were not allowed in our bedrooms. After several nights of no sleep, the nurses must have felt sorry for me. I was allowed to lie on the couch in the lounge watching the TV until I fell asleep. After two weeks, I was able to go to sleep by reading. One of the regulations regarding TV was we were only allowed to watch recovery-based movies or programs during the week. I can't tell you how many times I watched "The Betty Ford Story" over and over. I never did, however, see the ending since I fell asleep just as she was being admitted to a Navel Recovery Hospital in Florida!

Advice from BFC on how to fall asleep was to drink chamomile tea before bedtime. Apparently, the tea binds with a specific receptor in the brain that initiates sleep naturally. We all had been using some type of sedative to sleep. However, now we were on our own. We would take as much of the tea from the cafeteria as we were allowed—so many "tea parties" late at night! Unfortunately, if I was lucky enough to fall asleep, I would wake up within a couple hours needing to use the bathroom. I would need to repeat this entire process again.

My roommate was another story. She was a smoker and would save all her cigarette butts in her drawer. She was a chain smoker, and once her cigarettes were gone, there was no way of purchasing any more. Our room reeked of cigarette butts, and she had the most horrendous productive cough. She smelled rotten is the only word to describe her odor. My comment to my therapist was she will die from lung cancer before alcohol addiction. I found out later she passed away from lung cancer two months after leaving the center.

This was also around the time of the Monica Lewinsky and President Clinton fiascoes. I remember my mother telling me she loved the color of Monica's lipstick. Mom had her names on several waiting lists at local department stores to be called if the shade became available. We could only watch the news during the weekend, and then there was only one TV. Phone privilege was based on seniority. The new person on the block was left with phone privileges during the night.

The only way men and women could be together was during co-ed AA meetings, which met twice a day. This was imparted due to Elizabeth Taylor's rehab romance with Larry Fortensky. On the upside, Liz

(Taylor) donated a complete exercise gym we were required to attend daily for ninety minutes. One of the exercises we did was step aerobics. In the last couple of days, I finally mastered this activity. Everyone in the class gave me a standing ovation! I have no sense of rhythm.

One big issue to me was no caffeine at all! And yet, ninety-five percent of the women were smokers. When I brought this issue up, I was told, "Betty hates smoking" however she made the statement that no one would come to BFC if smoking was not allowed. Add to my other symptoms, one massive headache. I went to the dining hall to check out tea, all caffeine-free.

Every Saturday, we went as a group to the Eisenhower Hospital for an AA speakers' meeting. AA meetings always have real coffee at the meetings. Disappointed again. That was the time I scraped the chocolate frosting off several donuts. Could the frosting be caffeine-free, too? There was one bright spot, however. While we were at the Eisenhower hospital, one of the guys was able to sneak into the kitchen and stuff all of the pockets in his cargo pants with pre-packaged real coffee. We brewed a pot in our lounge. People say you cannot tell the difference between caffeine-free and caffeinated coffee, but the two smell completely different when brewing. That pot of coffee was gone in a matter of seconds. Several girls said they were going to continue to be caffeine-free when they coined out.

Me? Coffee is a legal high. During one of my last days, a fellow confidant gave me a can of Pringles' potato chips. She said they were from one of the guys who knew I liked coffee. As I took the can, I notice how heavy it felt. Going to my room, I opened the container and out slid a small instant coffee jar—real coffee. I would make myself a cup of real coffee every morning until I left. I almost felt guilty for drinking a cup, almost.

We had several lectures on not drinking at the airport. I later heard several girls stopped at a liquor store before ever arriving at the airport. I was just thrilled to order two cups of coffee as my beverage on the flight home. Betty Ford told her story, and we were given a copy of her book. I had the best intentions of never using again. My therapist tried to talk me into going into a four-month inpatient program when I arrived home. I reluctantly agreed to an outpatient program in Grand Rapids since I would be going back to my office job. I was also encouraged to go to ninety AA meetings in ninety days. My comment: "Maybe I can do two meetings a week." The bottom line—I lasted twelve days without using. That comes out to $1200 a day. I never wanted to commit to any suggestions completely. I would have saved myself and my family a lot of grief and money.

Additionally, Kristin flew out to BFC and stayed for an entire week, which was Family Week. I was so proud of her. She became even more critical, though, as she received some tools to help her deal with me and my continuing use.

Chapter Ten

MY FLIGHT BACK to Grand Rapids was uneventful. I was content to drink my caffeinated coffee.

I did not take the advice of BFC and go into a long-term treatment center for four months. BFC told me health-care people need more structure. However, I did my half-ass commitment and signed up for the Health Professional Recovery Program (HPRP), which is run by the state of Michigan. I self-reported to this company which would allow me to continue to work as a nurse. To be honest, I really didn't know what I was committing to. I just wanted to "coin out" of Betty Ford.

When I returned to Grand Rapids, I learned more about HPRP. I had forty-eight hours to sign consents or my nursing license would be pulled. My requirements were: 1) at minimum three AA meetings a week, 2) admit myself to a long-term treatment center for four months or outpatient three times a week, 3) every Monday an hour-and-a-half group therapy session consisting of all health-care people, 4) every Thursday a meeting for nurses only, 5) a weekly consultation with the addictionologist and CEO of the center, and 6) an hour of continuing education every Saturday morning.

Every morning I was required to call a phone number of a local lab to check if it was my day to go in for a urine drop. My "color" was purple. If the day's color was purple, I was ordered to report to a lab. If I did not show up at the lab, HPRP considered the urine positive. After two positive urines, I was out of the program, and my nursing license would be pulled. This program went on for three years. It was not cheap.

As I said earlier, I chose the "easier, softer way" for follow-up treatment, deciding on the outpatient option. My logic was I would be able to work and be a mother to my daughters.

I committed to outpatient treatment program. (This is the same treatment center that was suggested to me by BFC for four months). Outpatient and inpatient "students" met in the waiting room at eight o'clock every mornings. As I sat in that room, I watched as the inpatient clients walked in and took a seat. I noticed they were laughing and having a good time. I remember looking at them and thinking *I know I am going to end up being an inpatient.*

Chapter Eleven

MY LAST APPEARANCE as a nurse under the influence was at the "weekly nurses' meeting." People in this meeting were either inpatient, outpatient, or graduates of the treatment center. My speech was slurred as I checked in. The shirt I wore was not buttoned correctly; one shoe untied. Michelle, another nurse in recovery and today my BFF, sat next to me and said, "Gail, we would like you to give a urine sample. We think you are using."

Most people would deny being under the influence but not me. "Yes, I have been using. Do you still need a urine sample?"

Michelle was the first nurse I met who had a history of calling in her own medications to a pharmacy. I remember the first time we met. It was at the "weekly nurses' meeting." I told her I thought I was the only nurse who every called pharmacies. Her response, "No, we are everywhere!"

That ended my outpatient program and began the inpatient stay. I drove home. I remember looking for any pills I might have hidden, like a final send-off. Occasionally I would find a drug in my car under the front seat; however, I would look at it as a treat—a piece of candy and pop it in my mouth. Abby was living in New York City going to school. I called her to tell her my plan of being inpatient. She was very short with me. I can't blame her. I had indeed told her many times I was done using. Kristin was just out of high school and would stay in our condo. My parents lived about a mile away, also in Hudsonville. My mom was so happy I was going to be in treatment. She cried and cried. I am so thankful I was clean eleven years before she passed.

This is sad to say, but I believe losing my job of eighteen years was what it took to wake me up. How sad for my children.

Before I could be admitted into the inpatient program, I did a five-day stay at the same local hospital where I had previously stayed for detox. I drove myself. I was given some medication to detox, but the withdrawal was nothing like I had felt at BFC. After my third day, the detox medication was discontinued. I remember going to the nurse's station stating they forgot to give me all of my meds. I was informed that was it, the end. Okay, I tried. I just had to accept this.

My five days inpatient detox had ended. Since I drove to the hospital, I assumed I could go back to Hudsonville, pack my clothes, sheets, towels, and bathing necessities…everything I might need for the summer session as an inpatient which was May through August. I would not be going home for several weeks. My thinking was so far from recovery. When going back to get my belongings, I would make one, last, thorough, search for any pills or beer that may still be hidden. Imagine my surprise when the addictionologist would not allow me to drive by myself. The nurse on staff would be riding with me. Okay, so be it.

I arrived at my inpatient apartment around eight o'clock at night. Four women shared a two-bedroom, one bath apartment. I remember standing just inside the kitchen. They were watching the movie *Pin Head*. That's about all I remember of that night.

What am I doing here? I don't belong here. I don't want to be here.

There were two apartments for women, and three flats for men. We stayed on the northwest side of Grand Rapids. I was not familiar with that area, but it didn't take long to learn. It was near the East Beltline and Alpine. I was required to go to an AA meeting every day and attend church weekly. Several AA meetings were held at "The West Coast Club" which is a leading organization providing support meetings and fellowship for those fighting addictions. Every Friday the "No First Drink" meeting was held in Room H. It seems as though it was yesterday when I raised my hand to make a statement. I was told I should be pushing myself out of my comfort zone, something very difficult for me. I just knew I had nothing any one in that room wanted or needed to hear me say. My announcement was, "This is my third day of being sober."

To my surprise everyone in the room applauded. Wow, I looked around the room and everyone was smiling and genuinely happy for me. The last person to speak during the hour meeting thanked me for reminding her when she made a similar statement fifteen years ago.

Today I can honestly say I enjoy going to AA meetings. At first, I went because I was either in treatment or my sponsor told me to go. When not in treatment, I remember trying to come up with excuses—snow storm, I felt sick, the car wouldn't start, etc. Soon I realized even if I did not want to go, I always felt better after a meeting. It's kind of like exercising. I never really have a desire to go, although I always feel healthier and more positive about myself when I do go.

When I was still fairly new as an inpatient I was not to be alone for the first two weeks. Mother's Day was the first Sunday of my stay. I know Abby was fed up with my "attempts" to stop drinking. She did, however, still call to say she loved me. That call meant so much to me. I remember telling myself this time must be different, that I would do whatever I am told. The addictionologist told me one out of twenty in our group would "make it." I kept that in my memory.

One of my classmates had an appointment in Detroit on Mother's Day. Since I was not allowed to be by myself, I rode up and back with her. She was a doctor from California. She was trying to get a disability due to her alcohol addiction. I did not know her; but she was my roommate in my apartment. I was not feeling well. I wanted to stay home in bed. The drive from Grand Rapids to Detroit is a little over two hours. We stopped in Greektown, Detroit, for dinner. That was one of my first meals without alcohol. I always had a beer with my meals—what a long day. Several weeks later, she went back to California for a wedding. She relapsed, lost her medical license, and never came back to the treatment center. A short time later, we heard she had died.

The following morning, I allowed myself extra time to apply my makeup just right. I had an appointment the following week for a haircut back home, but I guess that would have to wait since home passes were not allowed during the first three weeks in rehab.

After glancing in the mirror before leaving the apartment, I felt as good as I could in this situation. I believed if I looked all put together, I was all together. That same day I recall my first group therapy session began. I was asked to give one of my long-range goals, to which I answered, "Growing my bangs out."

After all, I was here for a minimum of four months. My therapist asked if I often use humor as a defense, and I replied, "Yes, pretty much so."

Unfortunately, he did not find this comment humorous. The following week my assignment was quite simple. Since I was concerned about how I looked, I could not wear any makeup nor wash my hair for several days. I always took pride in good skin care. I have to say, no matter how intoxicated I was, I always managed to drag myself to the bathroom, cleanse my face, and apply night cream. I found the following morning to be uncomplicated along with less stress. I experienced a new meaning to the phrase lousy hair days. My days in rehab advanced to weeks, which moved forward into months.

On my last day, I was asked if I was satisfied with my growth. My response was, "Yes, it is incredible how quickly one's bangs grow in four and a half months."

Chapter Twelve

I WAS IN GROUP therapy, when my therapist, began the session by saying there was a person in the room she was very concerned with... someone who was not taking recovery seriously. I looked around the room, wondering who it must be. To my surprise, she said, "Gail."

Me? Why me? For the past several years, she reminded me that I never wholly accepted suggestions given to help me stop. Another fact was I did not look like your typical addict. I appeared to be too innocent. She said that was one of the reasons for my past ten years of using. She asked me what I hoped to learn this time.

"To learn more about the disease process."

She told me there was no more to learn. It was my time to take recovery seriously.

I remember a male resident named Todd. We went into treatment the same day. I could have listened to his stories all day. One of his best was, "Fishing while Drinking." He was in a small boat with a motor. Due to his drinking, he became unsteady. With the engine running, he fell into the water, only to see the motorboat turning around and heading right for him. He did manage to get out of the way. And maybe I see the humor in situations that are not funny, however, even our therapist could not help but laugh at that story.

Since I was I was inpatient during the summer of 1999, many of the guys wore shorts that were just too short, if you know what I mean. My solution to this situation was simple. Always sit next to the person with short shorts, not across from them in the circle.

Every morning the four of us in our apartment would "watch" each other take the medication and swallow the pill. We then had to document this on a card which would be submitted every week. This may sound ridiculous; however, alcoholics and drug addicts can be very devious. If someone would not swallow the Antabuse, they may be planning to sneak down to the store and buy alcohol. This is precise as one of my roommates did so on my third day. I think she took advantage of me being new. To make a long story short, she rode her bike to the closest liquor store and purchased a bottle of vodka. She tested positive for alcohol the following day. I learned my lesson. I was told that I was partially to blame because I did not verify that she swallowed the pill. Well, I don't know about that; however, that situation never occurred again.

When one was a newbie, many of the group events were directed toward that person. There were two groups. One was more aggressive than the other. I was in the more subdued group. I do not consider myself an aggressive person. I was asked to write my "losses" on the board at the front of the room. Since I am such a poor speller, I wondered if one of my friends could write as I spoke.

It took me a few minutes to understand what my therapist meant by losses. As she explained it to me, I understood that loss could be money, a death, an event, happiness, you get the picture. So, I began. I started with Kristin's health. She would always live with a neurological condition and later passed away from a glioblastoma; my divorce, loss of a husband, and the loss for my children not having a father in their life. The loss of Mike, my husband, to an illness; the loss of my health while taking care of him and the girls. I developed an ulcer and was in the hospital for three months; and the loss of my job I held for eighteen years. There is a saying, "I didn't lose my job; I gave it away." Also, I lost the respect and love of my daughters, Abby and Kristin. Thankfully, today we have a loving mother-daughter relationship. I am not justifying my addiction on losses, however I made poor choices in dealing with my life. Today I have many tools available to help me deal with life. Drugs and alcohol are not an option.

While in patient, I attended weekly Caduceus Meetings. Remember, this is the group of health-care professionals I went to over eight years ago. At the time, I just wanted to get out of that meeting and never go back. Well, there I was, back in this same group with thirty-five addicts and alcoholics. In that first meeting, I introduced myself by saying, "My name is Gail Mitcavish, alcoholic addicted nurse from Hudsonville."

After the introduction, people would give a short summary of their week. If they had a problem, they would ask for time. Or if the doctor felt like someone should tell their story, he would give them an opportunity. After going around the room, one of the last doctors to check in was the same one who, eight years ago, asked if I felt I was better than the rest of the group. I had lied to him about my using, sleeping, etc.

"I was wondering if you were going to resurface. It took eight years, and here you are. I am so thankful you are still alive." I believe I started crying.

It's funny how things work out, sometimes. I received $1,200.00 back from the drug company that manufactured Ativan, my all-time favorite. Several pharmaceutical companies overcharged consumers millions of dollars in higher prescription prices. I had paid cash for this drug because I didn't want my insurance company to track my many "scripts." Ironically, the reimbursement went toward my treatment!

During another Caduceus meeting, a doctor shared he would ask his patients to bring their medication bottles to their appointments which would give him an opportunity to go over their meds with them. He would pour several pills into his hand, telling the patient he was making sure they were taking the correct prescription, but palming some of the pills in his hand and placing them into his pocket. Many health-care professionals in these meetings admitted to going through people's medicine cabinets looking for prescription bottles and an opportunity to take some pills home with them.

Depression is often intertwined with addiction. Depression can be such a powerful emotion. After several weeks, one of the men was late getting to our first class. A couple of the guys went to his apartment and found he had hung himself.

A second incident occurred during my four-and-a-half-month stay. A pharmacist went home to Holland, Michigan, for the weekend. He mentioned he was going for a walk along Lake Michigan. When he didn't come home, his family went looking for him. He had shot himself in the dunes along the lake.

Addiction is such a baffling and cunning, yet powerful, disease.

Permission to leave the campus had to be granted each time someone would go home for a weekend, meet someone for coffee at a coffee shop, or keep an appointment. We were being taught accountability. Specifically, I learned to be accountable for my behavior and to care deeply about how my actions affected those I loved. I even was required to get permission to meet with my minister at a restaurant across the street. Being accountable is ongoing.

Every Wednesday was Family Day. The fact that my family was only several miles away guaranteed them to be present every week. Kristin and my mom came every Wednesday. The sessions were always fascinating, seeing the dynamics of families. Kristin always had some interesting "stories" to bring up.

One of my lessons on being accountable involved one of my condominium neighbors. During the winter, I had hidden some beer outdoors next to the air conditioning unit. That spring Kristin had found it. As she placed it in the trash, my neighbor saw her.

"Getting rid of the beer before your mother finds it?"

Kristin just laughed and let him assume the beer was hers. This was, of course, "discussed" on Family Day. It was decided I would talk with my neighbor that weekend and take responsibility for the beer. I very seldom spoke with him so you can imagine his surprise when I knocked on his door. In so many words, I stated, "The beer you saw the other day was not Kristin's but mine. I am in a long-term treatment program for drugs and alcohol, and want to be honest with you."

He looked at me with a blank stare and began talking about his son's new promotion at a large company in Chicago. I thanked him for his time. That conversation took place for Kristin, not him. The subject was never brought up again during the eight years we were neighbors.

Another one of my roommates lived nearby. Her family came just as often as mine. Every Family Day, her youngest son would ask the same question.

"May I ask my mom a question?"

The therapist would reply, "Of course."

He then proceeded to tell the story we had heard over and over. "My mom took my two brothers and me to the movie. Mom settled us in with popcorn and pop, and she went to see another movie. "

We all knew the end of the story. Mom had brought a bottle of alcohol with her and had fallen asleep/passed out while watching her movie. The children were unable to awaken her. They called their dad. He drove to the theater, found his children, and left without waking his wife. Situations similar to this were all too familiar to all of us. I felt uncomfortable and so sad. I looked back at the many times I placed my children's safety at risk. I think about the many times I drove drunk with them in the car. I remember them crying, begging me to stop driving, especially in the winter when the roads were icy. I am so fortunate I was not the cause of an accident or injuring myself but more importantly, innocent people.

One of my favorite AA meetings was in Grandville on Wednesday night, at eight o'clock. I called it the "Old Timers Meeting." Most of the members were men who had many years of sobriety and a great deal of wisdom. As mentioned earlier, one of their favorite words of wisdom was the phrase, "Show Me Don't Tell Me." This applied to me. I had to show Kristin I was serious this time and not just tell her. I had to earn that trust. It took many years for this trust to return but I knew at some point the trust would return.

While I attended the AA meeting, Kristin would go to an Al-Anon meeting in another room. She received so much support from those members. Al-Anon is a mutual support program for people whose lives have been affected by someone else's drinking. It was so crucial for Kristin to find the support. They helped her realize she could not make me stop drinking.

Another one of my accountability assignments involved contacting all twelve of my pharmacies where I called fictitious patient's medications in to be filled. When using drugs, I would go to the pharmacy, give the fake name, and walk out with these "scripts" called in under the doctors I worked for. To hold me accountable, my therapist opened her office, and I sat down at her desk. To my surprise, she also sat down and asked me if I knew why she was staying in the room. Could it be that she did not trust me to follow through with all the calls?

When the pharmacist answered the phone, I began, "I am in a long-term treatment center for drugs and alcohol." I went on to give the pharmacist the fake names. Some would ask for my name to which I politely said, "No."

Most said, "Congratulations, and I hope you do well."

Growing up, I was taught to tell the truth and not lie, but somehow lies entered my daily life. I found myself lying even when I didn't need to. The Big Book states the only alcoholics who can't stop drinking are those who cannot be honest. No addiction is without lies. No recovery is without the truth. This was made known to me over and over. It's something I worked very hard on. In AA, this is called rigorous honesty—telling the truth when it's easier to lie, sharing thoughts and feelings even when there may be consequences.

My faith was one of the first beliefs to leave me, and it took quite some time to return. I remember putting sticky notes around the apartment reminding me to pray. Being brought up in a "Christian" home and school, I found this odd.

I was nearing the end of my inpatient stay after four months when I stopped at a Walgreens to buy some candy. As I waited in line, I noticed a white pill lying on the counter. I had no idea what it was. It didn't look like candy, so in my mind, I thought it might be a mood-altering drug of some kind. When I stepped up to the counter, I scooped the pill up and put it in my pocket. My common sense returned while driving back to my apartment. Even if it was a pain pill, if I took it, the drug would show up in one of my many urine tests. I managed to throw the medication out the window. I remember sharing my actions with my roommate. She, of course, said it was my responsibility to bring this up in my group the following day, which I did. However, because of my actions, the addictionologist stated I would be staying another two weeks. Bummer...

I continued to take the two medications that helped me "not take a drug or drink." I amazed myself when I began to realize I could live without feeling high. I also knew a cold beer always tasted the best when I was hungry. I made a point of keeping a snack with me at all times. A favorite time for drinking was on my drive home from work. Well, since I did not have a job nor a driver's license, that temptation was gone. Since another favorite drinking time was on the deck of a restaurant, I did not sit on an outside patio for at least one year—no pop in a frosted mug, no drinking out of a can. I watched very little football on TV.

Kristin told me on Family Day, she hated Sundays because of my drinking with football. Drinking was involved in every part of my life. If I was unable to drink in a situation, I would take pills. Wow!

Just a few facts about the girls I shared my apartment with. One purchased a gun one night on Division Street in Grand Rapids, where vandalism often occurs. One biked to a local liquor store, bought vodka, and proceeded to drink while on Antabuse. One continued to take the medication, Ativan. I wondered why she always seemed so relaxed. She later said it was prescribed for her heart condition. Ativan is the drug that was so hard for me to get off of while at the Betty Ford Center. One said, "I have the Lord to help me stop." One was a crack head who took everything not nailed down out the door, and one relapsed while attending a wedding in California. She later passed away. (I believe I mentioned this earlier.)

Chapter Thirteen

AS THE END of my treatment was nearing, I began to get anxious. *Where will I work? I am forty-eight years old and lost my job due to using drugs and alcohol. Who would be interested in employing me?*

The addictionologist spoke with the office where I last worked and asked if they would consider hiring me back. They said, "No." Okay, I didn't blame them. Deep inside, I knew it would be better for me to start at a new job. The doctors I had worked with were just the best. They were never too busy to answer any questions a nurse might have had. Family always came first, and they had the best sense of humor and were always sensitive to the needs of their patients.

Applying for a new job was scary. My role at Hematology had been for the past eighteen years. I could have done it with my eyes closed. I knew this new job would be different, though. The state of Michigan was holding my nursing license. I would be signing a three-year contract. Also, I was required to be honest and tell my interviewer my history. I also wanted to work in a "safe environment." So, my main priority was not to work around any mood-altering drugs.

One of the safe nursing positions was in kidney dialysis. The only medication on that unit would be Tylenol. My addictionologist arranged an interview for me at the dialysis unit in St. Mary's Hospital. I later found out there were two other nurses in recovery working at that center. My work history before my last job was excellent. I did not jump around from job to post.

Three nurses applied for this position, and I'm very thankful, they chose me. I spent several days "shadowing" a nurse. The unit was downtown in Grand Rapids—not a perfect area at that time. Plus, the patients lived in poverty and had virtually no health care before being on dialysis. At least half of the people in the thirty-six-chair ward were in wheelchairs. It was an eye-opener for me. I was very thankful to have that job, but I did not realize all I was responsible for learning. Well, at least I had a clear mind and a desire to learn.

My training would involve flying to St. Louis for two weeks. My sponsor and I looked up meetings close to the hotel. I planned on going to three AA meetings per week. My visit would be my first time out of town since I stopped drinking. I remember many people who relapsed while out of town away from their home group, away from people who knew them, and friends who would recognize their abnormal behavior. Well, I'm happy to say I did well! Others went out after class, but I had no problem saying, "No." I finally realized my most important phrase to remember: "No first drink!" But look how long it took me to finally, "get it."

In one of the last classes, our instructor called some of us to review the incorrect answers we had given on the previous exam—

people who could use a little boost in their final grade. Yup, our teacher called my name. Now, mind you, our names were called because we had answered a question incorrectly. She was giving us a second chance to get a better grade. She read the problem to me. There were four answers to choose from, and I had chosen a wrong answer. She asked me to reread the question and make a choice. After looking over the answers, my statement to her was, "I'm going to stick with my answer."

OMG, I must be crazy! I guess it's good to know that some things never change.

There were two nurses in recovery, who worked with me in the clinic, they both relapsed. The other employees would come to me if they suspected one might be drinking or taking pills. I later said that I felt I must have had a big "A" on my forehead for "the alcohol police!" I could do nothing except talk with the coworker, then call the supervisor, and take them off the floor. When one is using in a situation like this, we never believe anyone can tell...so wrong. They both lost their jobs. The second nurse was drunk when she came in to pick up her check. She then locked herself in the bathroom. When she finally came out of the restroom half an hour later, she was more alert. She proceeded to leave the building, get in her car, and drove home. The second nurse did have some cognitive testing done. The diagnosis was a "wet brain," which is brain damage due to alcohol consumption. Neither one ever worked in nursing again.

Starting a new job at the age of forty-eight was easier than I thought. Most dialysis patients did not have a primary care physician. The nephrologist took on that role. I was happy to see a nephrologist was one of the doctors who visited the clinic. I had met her many years before. She was a friend with the hematologist from my previous job. She asked me how I was doing. I told her I was doing well, and I remember not feeling so ashamed. Somewhere in the past six months, I had learned gratitude for where I was. Going to meetings and hanging out with people in recovery made it easy to lose sight of how few people stay sober. Staying sober is challenging. Recovery is so precious. Sixty percent of the people who are treated for addiction relapse during their first year. I couldn't have done this without my mother and daughters, my biggest fans.

While working at St. Mary's dialysis clinic, the doctor mentioned she also went to Zeeland, Michigan, and was the director at that center. I lived in Hudsonville at that time, and driving to Zeeland would be much easier for me, not to mention the type of patient would be less complicated since most of them had primary care physicians and a strong family core. Unlike the Grand Rapids clinic, they would walk in, weigh themselves, and check their temperatures.

I accepted the job, and it took a little time for me to get used to the more independent patients. One of them, Lily, was happy to have someone do everything for her. I was on my hands and knees, putting her boots on and buttoning her coat. One of the nurses said, "Gail, you don't have to dress her!"

"Right." I laughed.

I was instructed to find a sponsor. I asked a nurse who could be pretty demanding. She was not afraid to tell me if I was wrong. I had made poor decisions for a long time. I needed someone who would hold me accountable for my actions.

I remember shortly after "graduation," I was home making a to-do list. I had not been home for four and a half months. I also did not have a job, which made me feel anxious. My sponsor called me and asked what I was doing. I told her creating a to-do list. She wondered how long my list was. I counted the twelve entries. She said to pick two and put the list away! Okay then…

Around this time, I sponsored a young nurse who was still in-patient. We met at a nurses' meeting. I worked with her for several months. She seemed to be accountable. However, before a meeting, she came running up to me, "I'm meeting a guy for coffee." She then asked me to lie to the counselor and say she didn't feel well.

My response: "I will give you fifteen minutes to call the supervisor in charge and tell him your plans. If you don't, I will. And since you have no respect for me, you can also find another sponsor." That was another reward of sobriety…being honest and saying what I think. Keep it simple.

Chapter Fourteen

MOM WAS EIGHTY-TWO when she began to have health issues. One of the signs we knew something was not right was her lack of interest in shopping. Mother was a die-hard shopper, always has been and always will be. We noticed she was doing more shopping on QVC. However, when Abby suggested we visit her and Gus in Chicago and go shopping, she hesitated for a moment and said no.

"I'm just too tired."

My mom was being treated for hypertension for as long as I could remember. Her blood pressure was well-controlled for years. But then, many of the medications caused her to have side effects: a cough, extreme fatigue, and shortness of breath.

One medication would lower it so much she had difficulty walking, while others had no impact on keeping her blood pressure down. Mom was loved by everyone who knew her. She was so much fun, always on the go. So, when she had a lot of complaints, I knew something was "going on."

I had picked her up on a Sunday morning. We were on our way

to church. I came to a four-way stop and started to turn into the church's driveway.

"Boy, I don't feel right," Mom said.

I asked her what she meant. "I'm having pain in my chest," she said.

I parked the car and asked her if I should call 911 or if it was okay for me to drive her to the emergency room (ER). She didn't feel there was a need to call 911. Mom spent several hours in the ER that day. My brother and sister met us there. I remember the doctor asking her if she had pain on her skin, in the area of her heart. He stated sometimes shingles begins before the sores appear as "chest pain." I remember dismissing this idea almost as soon as he mentioned shingles. Heart problems ran in her family. Her father and brother both had heart attacks.

After ruling out any acute issues, the doctors ordered a cardiac workup. She was on Coumadin, a blood thinner, for years due to an irregular heartbeat. The doctor felt a heart catheterization was necessary. Our family agreed, and the procedure was scheduled for a couple of weeks in the future. Blood work was scheduled. As we waited for the planned test, I couldn't believe what Mom showed me. She indeed developed shingles in the exact area over her heart and around to spine. The pain was so severe, pain medication did not completely stop it.

The doctor still felt a heart catheterization was the right choice to proceed. Mom went off the Coumadin for a couple of days. Just before the procedure began, a nurse started an IV. Before she was wheeled out, she was given some Demerol to help her relax and help with the pain. I remember her saying, "Oh, my pain is gone. I haven't been without pain for so long."

At that moment, I realized how severe her pain was with the shingles. She was not a complainer. After the catheterization was finished, her doctor told us it would take three days to get the results. The heart catheterization was normal. So, the chest pain was from shingles. Meanwhile, she would require Heparin IM injections before going back on the oral Coumadin. Since I am the nurse in the family, I had no problem with this. She required lab work daily to make sure the blood thinner was adjusted correctly. Mom needed one more shot, and she would go back to the oral Coumadin.

I believe it was a Sunday. My brother received a call from one of Mom's neighbors. She had called him to tell him that Mom's Sunday paper was lying on her doorstep. It was already noon. I had just made sweet potatoes and put the oven on low. "Cook them low and slow," Mom always said. He called me and asked me to meet him at the condo. Something wasn't right. In my haste to get to my mom's place, I thought I was turning the oven off. Leaving the sweet potatoes in the turned-off range would allow them to cook slowly.

Well, I had not only left the oven on, but I also turned the oven temperature as high as it would go—just the opposite from off. When I reached the condo, my brother had already gone in and found Mom on the floor. She appeared to have been walking out of the bathroom and collapsed. The doctor later said he believed she had a blood clot that lodged in her heart. All the events seemed to be going in slow motion.

I had been gone from my apartment, approximately three hours. Kristin was at work. As I turned the corner when returning home, I saw two fire trucks in my parking lot. *Wow, what is going on?* After walking up two flights of stairs to my apartment, I realized the smoke was coming from my place. A fireman had knocked the door down with an ax and was standing in the doorway without a door. Another fireman was holding my nine by thirteen-inch pan. Yup, there was my pan of sweet potatoes. I have to say they appeared to be small hockey pucks, black.

"It appears you turned the oven up to five hundred degrees and left."

As I walked to the office, I remember mumbling something like, "I'm sorry, we found my mother on the floor dead." I told them I would pay for any loss not covered by insurance. They never gave me a bill. The damage was smoke. Abby and Gus would be driving up from Chicago and staying with me during Mom's funeral. The smoke smell lingered a long, long time. It was quite a while before I made sweet potatoes again.

My belief is in life after death. There is never a right time to die. I thought Mom fell to the floor and tried to crawl to the phone for help. I did not wish to picture her last moments struggling. A couple of days later, I just had to ask my brother how he found her.

"She was just as you saw her on the floor." He had not moved her. This little bit of information gave me some comfort. One more note: an order from QVC arrived the next day for Mom—hot pink, cropped pants! That was our mother!

Chapter Fifteen

I WAS LEARNING to take responsibility for my recovery. During Family Day, this subject was brought up: "I hope my brother does not expect our family drinking habits to change because of him."

The therapist asked, "Has he asked you to change?"

"No," was the response.

You see, my choice to drink or not to drink has nothing to do with others. I have learned if I am going to be around alcohol, I will always drive myself. If I feel uncomfortable in a situation, I will always have the option of escape.

In my first three years in recovery, my license was held by the state of Michigan. I was not allowed to work around narcotics. (Could I not be trusted?) I was required to have a worksite monitor. A person would fill out monthly reports based on my working performance. I have a great deal of respect for nurses who take this position. I was thankful to my addictionologist, for helping me find my job in dialysis.

After my three-year contract with the state expired, I still attended the nurses' meeting and the Caduceus meetings. They both have a great deal of knowledge and experience to share.

Last, but not least, I had a monthly visit with my addictionologist. He advised me to have no new relationships for one year. Alcoholics can hardly handle their own lives, let alone someone else's, too. Next, he advised me to keep a plant alive for one year, and lastly, keep a pet alive for one year. Only then would I be ready to try a relationship!

Regaining my daughter's trust would not come so easy. When I was still drinking, Kristin would ask me if I was going to drink while she was gone. My answer would be, "No," but I always would be drunk when she came home. We set up some ground rules. If she wanted me to check in with her, I would, and she would check in on me at any time. I told her I would do everything in my power to not drink or drug again.

Restoring trust with my mom was an ongoing process. My sister, brother, and his wife were planning on driving down to Nashville for the weekend. For some reason, the plans fell through. I stopped at Mom's house on my way home from work to tell her we would not be going. Her response to me was, "I know why your plans fell through."

"Really, why was that?" I couldn't imagine what she was going to say.

"Because you were going to drink during your time away."

I'm not sure what my response was to her, but it upset me. I said a quick goodbye and got into my car, ready to drive home. I decided to go back and talk with my mom. I knew if I did not respond to her comment, I would regret it. I explained to her how much her comment hurt me. I was seven years sober. The length of time was not even the issue. If I wanted to drink, I didn't need to drive out of town to do that. I could do no more than I was doing every day to prove this to her. I know she was shocked at my response and started to cry. I hugged her and told her how much I loved her. However, it was the right thing to say and the right time to say it.

My mom was a saint. She was what you might call "a natural born worrier!" I tried to never give her or Kristin any reason to think I might relapse.

Chapter Sixteen

MY MOTHER'S DEATH was unexpected; however, I was relieved she did not hear the news when my daughter, Abby, was diagnosed with appendix cancer. Two years after Mom passed away, Abby and Gus moved from Chicago to Houston, Texas. Gus grew up in Katy, Texas, and he missed his family, especially his two nephews, who were four and five years old.

I would miss visiting them in Chicago. My mom, Kristin, and I would often take the train out of Holland, Michigan, or make the three-hour drive. Abby had moved to New York right after high school graduation. She attended college there and lived in Manhattan for seven years. After going through the 911 terrorist attacks in New York City, she decided to move to Chicago, where she met Gus.

They moved to Houston in November of 2010. I remember when Abby told me they were moving. "Houston, what is in Houston?'" I asked her. Little did I know, Houston was where she should be living.

In July 2012, she called me at work to tell me she did not feel well—had pain in her lower abdomen. I suggested she call her primary care provider and to let me know what they said. After one hour went by, I decided to call Abby. "What did the nurse or doctor say?"

"I didn't call them. I sent them an email."

"Abby, hang up this phone and call the office. It would be best if you talked with someone. It's Friday afternoon, and you should do something now. And call me back."

Well, it turns out it was her appendices. Her primary care physician was in the medical center. She was seen in his office and carried her films (X-Rays) across the street to St. Luke's Hospital. The surgery was uneventful. When she called me the next day, I said, "Hi honey, are you home?"

"No, Mom, it's cancer." She started to cry. I felt so helpless. Plus, she was there alone. Gus was on his way to pick her up.

Often, I seem to have a hard time saying nothing. My mouth seemed to act independently, blabbering on autopilot. I remember hanging up the phone after talking with her. *I just need to talk with Gus and ask if he has any additional information. Maybe Abby doesn't know or remember all the information the doctors must have said.*

I called Gus. He was just driving into the parking garage to take Abby home. I asked him if he knew any more about what was scheduled or planned for treatment. Well, not only did he not have any additional information, Abby had not told him about cancer. She wanted to tell him face to face. I felt so bad. In fact, she mentioned this the other night when we were talking about that time in her life. Well, I don't care for the statement, "It is what it is." But that sums it up.

We purchased tickets for Kristin and me to fly to Houston for Abby's surgery in just a few days. I remember thinking I was so thankful I was sober to handle this situation in our lives. Gus's father picked us at the George W. Bush airport north of Houston, Texas. We stayed with Abby and Gus, who had just moved into a new two-bedroom apartment. By just moved, I mean one week. Abby was discharged two days after we arrived. Kristin and I were going to be in Houston for one week. We helped her get around, did laundry, and went to the grocery store.

Their computer had not been connected yet due to the move. The day after the hookup, Gus was at work; it was early morning, and I awoke to hear Abby crying in her bedroom. I went into her bedroom and found her under her blankets, saying, "I don't want to die."

I looked at the computer screen, and she was reading about appendiceal cancer. I tried to console her as best I could. What do you say to your daughter in this situation? I did all I could, which was hold her and tell her how much I loved her, and that we would get through this.

I can remember as though it was yesterday when Kristin was three years old. She had just been diagnosed with NF and optic nerve glioma. Her ophthalmologist told me the same thing. As I faced him from across his desk, he looked straight at me and said, "You will get through this, Gail. I know right now that doesn't seem possible. But you will."

He was right. We had Kristin another twenty-nine years.

While we were in Houston, a second, more aggressive surgery was scheduled a month away. This first surgery was only to remove her appendices and obtain a biopsy. Her follow-up visit with her surgeon was scheduled three days after we flew home. I knew we all needed to meet with her doctor before Kristin and I left for Michigan.

The next day we made a call to her doctor's office. I asked if we could come in to talk in the next couple of days. The receptionist stated, "He does not have any appointments available."

I asked if she had a few minutes to listen to what I had to say. I explained I was Abby's mom, and my daughter, Kristin, and I had tickets to fly back to Michigan in two days. We had questions we needed to ask. She placed us on hold, which seemed like an eternity. Thoughts that came back to me were being in the same situation at my previous job when the doctors I worked with would give up their lunch hour to talk with patients who were in the same position as we were now. Could she please ask him if we could have just a few moments to talk?

"He has time tomorrow during our lunch hour."

"Thank you so much!"

He transferred Abby to MD Anderson, and they would take over her care. She was the third patient he ever had with this diagnosis. He answered all the questions we had, and we thanked him for his time.

We came back to Houston in four weeks. Her doctor at MD Anderson performed the second surgery, a two-hour operation. Abby was in the recovery room when the doctor came to talk with us. Gus,

Kristin, and I were escorted into a small conference room. I do not believe I heard much after his first statement.

"Abby has tumors in her colon, stomach, liver, lung, and one of her ovaries."

I sat back in my chair. I think I just shut down. I couldn't even ask any questions. Poor Gus walked over to his dad and mom in the waiting room and started crying…such a long day.

Since MD Anderson is a teaching hospital, Abby decided to sign into a clinical trial. I again voiced my expert opinion, "Now is not the time to be heroic, Abby. Say you want the treatment with the best results."

Of course, she did not listen to me. The cancer was very slow-growing. She decided to enjoy her summer and schedule the subsequent surgery for the end of August. I couldn't believe what she was saying. Enjoy the summer? I would have planned it for the next day or the next hour if I could. Well, her doctor was okay with her choice. She gained a little weight and harvested a couple units of her red blood cells in the event she needed a blood transfusion during her surgery. The pre-surgical clearance test was scheduled. Back to Michigan for the summer. I thought August would never arrive.

I also found an AA meeting in the MD Anderson Hospital. This was great. It met twice a week and included many health-care people and others whose family or friends were patients. It was so convenient for me to be able to go to a meeting in the hospital. They often mentioned the fact that alcoholism is a chronic disease. A disease that is treatable but not without relapse and possible death.

MD Anderson was one of three hospitals in the United States that treated this cancer of the appendices. The treatment was very different from the traditional treatment. No IV chemotherapy, no radiation, no hair loss. The surgery would take at least ten to twelve hours. The doctors would make an incision from just below her rib cage and end several inches below her navel. They would start from the top and go through every part of her abdominal cavity, including all the organs. They would cut and remove every tumor they could see or feel— after which, they would cauterize any suspicious areas. Comparison would be made with recent MRIs. The last two hours of the procedure would involve filling her abdominal cavity with "heated chemotherapy" and sloshing it back and forth while on the operation table.

Gus's parents were lifesavers. They would bring their homemade Mexican meals to the hospital, and we would take the food up to the top floor, where there were several areas to eat overlooking the city of Houston. The food was delicious! His mom makes the most beautiful, best-tasting salad I have ever had! They are both such gracious and loving people. I am blessed to have them in my life.

I often thought about how thankful I was for my sobriety. There were many years when I was not there for my daughters. Sobriety is such a gift. Because I "hung around with the winners," I forget how many alcoholics don't make it. As I was told in treatment, one out of twenty would relapse, and many would never get back.

As I opened Abby's door to enter her hospital room, I watched

Abby and Gus as they appeared to be struggling with her bedpan. Something did not look right. It looked like they were working with an emesis basin instead of a bedpan. In fact, Gus had actually found a second emesis basin, thinking one was not adequate. I laughed so hard I almost cried. I did a little private duty nursing and helped them out.

Abby's prognosis was not good. Thirty percent lived for five years. This information made me consider moving to Houston. My mother was no longer living, which would have held Kristin and me back. There were so many factors to consider. The more Kristin and I talked, the more we felt it to be the right choice.

I knew this would be good, especially for Abby and Kristin. Historically, they had never gotten along. Abby had gone to college in New York City, which was actually a very healthy choice. This left Kristin to do everything in her power to stop me from drinking. Abby was so angry with me for drinking. I think she took it out on Kristin, and even though Kristin and I would visit her in Chicago, they had very little sister time. Abby was twenty-two, and Kristin was twenty when I finally stopped drinking.

Since Abby was currently being treated at MD Anderson and her follow-up care would continue there, after much prayer and contemplation, we finally made our decision to move. I worked for Dialysis Centers in Zeeland Michigan, and I found I could transfer from my center in Holland to Houston. Kristin worked at Dick Sporting Good's at the time.

Our family is not big—it's just my sister, her daughters, and my older brother and his wife and two children. Sure, there was Christmas and Thanksgiving and occasional get-togethers, but family would not deter us from moving.

Chapter Seventeen

I FLEW DOWN to Houston to check out some of the apartments and possibly nursing jobs available. I seemed to be burned out in working in dialysis for ten years so I was looking for something different. The first apartment we looked at was in the medical district of Houston.

"What is the apartment heated with I asked the manager?

After a slight pause, he said, "Electricity."

"Oh boy, electricity is so expensive to heat with. Why not gas?"

"Mom, we are in Texas. You are not going to need any heat."

Okay, I knew that, too. We found a two-bedroom apartment on the second floor around fifteen minutes from Gus and Abby... It was near the Houston NRG stadium. This location proved to be crazy out-of-control traffic during football season.

Kristin and I moved in April of 2013, six months after Abby's surgery. Transferring my nursing license proved to take some time. I believed I was transferring my Michigan LPN license to Texas, however, I was only showing Texas I had a current, up-to-date nursing license. My history of being in treatment and the three-year contract I had with Michigan had been destroyed, so my addiction history didn't impact potential employment. I soon found out Texas did not seem to do anything quick, simple, or cheap. Texas required a payment of $400 and taking a state nursing test. Most states only required filing a form online, and the information on my license was current and up to date. Here, I accepted a transfer from the dialysis company in Zeeland to a center in Houston. I was in class learning about the new dialysis machines when I was called out of the class. It was at that time it was discovered my license was not current in Texas. I was unable to work as a nurse until my request was transferred entirely.

Meanwhile, Kristin had decided she wanted to attend Houston Community College. She was interested in the certified nursing assistant (CNA) courses. Kristin had been in retail in Michigan and was ready for a change. We checked out the requirements, which included providing proof she was up to date on all her vaccinations. We went through every piece of paper in our business files. Kristin, of course, thought she was adopted since I had copies of all Abby's medical records from day one. The only way she was going to get into school was to get every required shot. That doesn't sound too difficult; however, one of the requirements was the Hepatitis B Vaccination series which would take a total six months. So we began the waiting game. I had never been without a job. I decided to focus on going to AA meetings and getting to meet new friends.

Kristin started working at Toys 'R' Us. I gave flu shots around the city since I was able to obtain a temporary license for four months. I was happy when I finally received my Texas nursing license and could begin my job in dialysis.

The machines at this center were different. After training on the new machines, I stated I did not feel comfortable working with patients. They said I was given the training I needed. Working in a new job is difficult but not feeling confident in what I was doing was the worst.

To make a long story short, I quit. In all my working career, I never quit a job or even considered. I just knew I could not work there without any more training. The fear I felt was overwhelming. I talked with the manager and asked him if I would qualify for unemployment. He said, "Yes." I would have quit if he had said, "No."

When I filed unemployment in Texas, the unemployment office informed me that I would be filing through Michigan and not Texas since I was a dialysis nurse in Michigan for the past ten years. After speaking with someone at the unemployment center, they suggested I check out the list of available legal counsels. To say I knew nothing about unemployment was putting it mildly. I was sixty-two and had always worked. My work history began at nine years of age "topping onions" in the muck. After giving my job history of the past several weeks, the state representative of Michigan informed me, "Oh wait, you live in Texas now? Well, unfortunately, you do not qualify for any assistance because of your location." Okay then!

My journey in obtaining unemployment continued. I do not even remember how many times my appeals were denied. I was so depressed during this time in my life. I waited for my nursing license in Texas to become valid and worked on getting my denied benefits.

I did obtain some legal advice from several lawyers, who were in my AA meetings. Most people give up. However, I was not like most people. I was so grateful for my recovery. If I may coin a phrase—my worst day sober far exceeds my best day drinking. I had found a great home group and firm friends in AA.

After my last appeal, the judge ruled I would be paid unemployment compensation retroactive from my first denial. It was also stated employers are successful in denying appealing unemployment more often than employees. I believed in my decision. I felt the dialysis patients were not safe under my care without more training. Yay!

It seemed as though our lives were settling into a more normal phase. I had my Texas nursing license. Abby worked full time and felt well. Her scans, which she had every four months, were stable. Kristin finally started her school since she had "all her shots!"

I interviewed for several jobs in health care. One was working as a nurse at the Harris County Correctional Center. Being sixty-two, I had enough common sense and realized that job wasn't going to work out for me. Another position was at Texas Children's Hospital. The hospital is one of the best in the country; however, just going from my car to the tram, to a bus, transferring to the right bus, and walking the last block would have been way too much for me. I chose to work for Grifols Plasma, one of the largest plasma companies worldwide.

The center I started at was thirteen miles from my home. That did not sound like too bad of a drive; however, the commute would take me from a six-lane expressway to a four-lane. Oh my, nearly every commute to and from work involved an accident of some kind. And then there was the rodeo and the Houston Texans—all in my commute to work. Speaking of the rodeo, I was comparing it to the Hudsonville Fair back home. The fair lasted for five days. Okay, I could deal with five days of crazy traffic, but when I was told the duration was three-and-a-half weeks, oh my! In fact, I believe the Houston Rodeo is one of the largest in the country. That's Texas for you!

I had worked for approximately two months when my manager called me into his office. He asked me if I was interested in working at a center that had just lost several nurses. It would only be for two weeks. Do I take a moment to say, "Let me think about it, or I'll get back to you, or even no"?

I hardly knew what I was doing at my center, let alone enough to help at another. My manager also said that center had a guard on duty full time due to the location and clientele. For some reason, I blurted out, "Yes, I can help." Why do I do that? I guess at my age, if I have not learned how to say, "I'll get back to you in the morning," I never will. But my decision to help at the other center was the right choice. I'm still there after eight years. This might not be the right way to say this, but I was the only white person there for a long time. The team is so much fun to work with, and the donors are the best. Very respectful. They have a great sense of humor. Everyone calls me Miss Gail! I love it.

Chapter Eighteen

I WAS SO PROUD of Kristin for following through on her desire to become a nursing assistant. Her schooling was a total of six months in class in addition to working at various nursing or retirement centers for hands-on training.

I can remember it as if it were yesterday, no this morning. I remember telling Kristin how she accomplished so many of the goals she had set for herself. She was excited to move to Houston, not only to be near her sister, but to start a new chapter in her life.

The sadness and emptiness I feel that her life was cut short are sometimes so overwhelming. These emotions can come over me so quickly. For example, at work, I can be reading several pages of information to a donor and somehow find myself thinking of Kristin while I am reading. We miss her so much. I have to regroup, push forward, and say a prayer.

Kristin had two tests she needed to pass before receiving her Texas CNA license. She always had difficulty with written tests. People with the diagnosis of NF often have learning disabilities. We drove out of the Houston city limits to a testing center with more accessible parking since I would go with Kristin and wait for her in the car. To my surprise, she aced the written test on the first try. They give you three attempts to pass, after the third try, you have to retake the six-month course if you don't pass. That was the last thing Kristin wanted.

Well, the hands-on final proved to be more of a problem than the first clinical test. She did not pass. Kristin's blood pressure reading for the "patient" was out of the range the teacher had gotten. She had two more tries. Did I mention you have to pay a fee for each test? Texas seems to have a price for every service provided. Even toll roads are everywhere! When I mention Michigan has zero toll roads, Texans are shocked.

Back to Kristin and the second test. We reviewed and practiced together with the requirements that were needed. We drove back to the testing center two weeks later. I took my place in the parking lot, again. I couldn't sit any longer while I waited, though. I walked around outside and prayed the whole time.

As I said a prayer, Kristin came out of the center.

Oh no! I could tell by Kristin's facial expressions it looked like another no-go. I felt so bad for her. She was such a sweet, loving person, tender-hearted and optimistic. When I look back at all the physical roadblocks she had overcome, the mean teasing she endured because she looked different, I was so proud of her. One more chance came. I told her, "You know this, Kristin," back in the parking lot for another try.

Kristin was the last one out the door. She slowly walked toward the car. *Please.* She looked at me and slowly shook her head. The car door opened, and she sat down.

"I passed!" She whipped out her certificate. That was such a "Kristin moment"!

I can almost cry thinking about it. Kristin's next challenge—sending out resumes. It seemed that in every position she applied for, there was the statement, "Must have experience." The only experience she had was in retail.

She did not let her lack of experience in health care stop her from sending her resumes out. Kristin had only one interview scheduled the first week. Sometimes one is all that is needed if it is the right one. She was hired at a senior citizen assisted living place called "The Hallmark." I still remember her first day. I came home from work at five o'clock and found Kristin sitting on the couch. I could tell something was wrong. I sat on the couch next to her. She said, "I don't know what to do, Mom."

I was distraught. *What was wrong?*

"I don't think I like my job."

Okay. I took a deep breath and said, "No one likes their job after the first day."

"Really?" she asked.

"Yes, Kristin." She was okay after that.

Abby continued to feel well. Her scans were every six months by now. Abby, Gus, and Kristin spent quality time together. Gus was employed in sales at a local brewery. He often would spend an evening in a local restaurant while Abby, Kristin, and I would eat dinner. Abby is vegan. Thank the Lord Gus enjoys a good, rare steak or a thick juicy hamburger! Once a week, Kristin and Gus would visit a different hamburger bar or restaurant. Abby was not invited since she was vegan. This competition was a fun way for the sisters to kid each other. I can't tell you how right our decision to move to Texas was.

I was so thankful for my recovery. I seemed to lose the insecurities that often made me drink in the first place. I can honestly say, "I love being sober."

Kristin grew to love her job. And the residents loved her. Many of them would wait for Kristin to help them to bed. They loved her positive personality.

Kristin met Barbara Bush several times as she visited one of her best friends who was a resident at "The Hallmark."

Now that Kristen worked full time, she wanted to buy a new car. Her old car had finally given up. It was an older, used Pontiac Grand Am when she bought it. Driving in Houston is something else…so much traffic! She needed a car she could rely on and settled on a Nissan Versa. I was so happy she could get a new car! She even purchased an extended warranty. She had purchased this on her previous car, and it had come in handy for several repairs. I co-signed the loan, and she was all set. Another accomplishment for her!

I feel so sad, guilt-ridden, and ashamed that I did not listen more to her physical complaints during this time period. I think I finally listened to her when she complained of weakness in her left arm. I believed she had pulled a muscle. We went to her primary care physician who took some time to diagnose her symptoms. She came home one night stating she was exhausted and must have hurt her back helping a patient. Then I sensed something was off…I don't think I will ever really forgive myself for not having figured it out sooner.

Chapter Nineteen

HER DOCTOR scheduled an MRI within a couple of days at Memorial Herman Hospital. Gus and Abby went with us to the consultation. The MRI showed a new tumor in her brain stem. Kristin had had tumors in this area of her brain since she was a child, which they believed were due to her NF. These had never increased in size. This tumor, however, was very different. They thought it to be a glioblastoma which is fast-growing and aggressive. We decided to go for a second opinion at MD Anderson. This is also where Abby had been treated for her appendix cancer.

I could not believe this! Kristin and I moved to Houston to support Abby two years earlier, and now Abby supported Kristin! When I worked at the hematology office in Grand Rapids, Kristin was five or six years old. The doctors once told me she had a twenty percent chance of developing cancer due to NF, which is a genetic disorder that can mutate into some types of cancer. Never in a million years had I foreseen this in our future.

The first doctor we saw at MD Anderson was a good fit. He was well-known in the treatment of NF. He talked about several options for treatment. One was monoclonal antibody drugs. Unfortunately, most of these types of treatments required a biopsy of the cancer tumor. Since Kristin's tumor was located in her brain stem, a biopsy was not possible. The brain stem has many essential functions, including regulating heart rate, breathing, sleeping, and eating. Surgery of any kind was out. That left radiation and some IV medications as treatment options that were used later. Kristin's prognosis was fifteen months. Of course, she was going to beat the odds!

We bought her a cane to help steady herself as she walked. She was unable to continue working. Kristin enjoyed her job so much—she loved working with the residents, but her body just couldn't endure much more.

In writing this, it seems more than four years since she passed. It was not long before her left arm and left leg were affected by the tumor. She finished the radiation treatments, which were five days a week for four weeks. Two weeks after the last radiation treatment, Kristin slept more, couldn't eat much, and had become more unsteady.

We went into the emergency room at MD Anderson, and the MRI showed although the tumor had decreased in size, there was also some swelling and inflammation. This was causing the symptoms Kristin was having. They decided to start her on a new treatment, an IV medication that would focus on the inflammation and hopefully shrink the area and give her more mobility with her left side. She was an inpatient for seven days, and the results were encouraging.

For the first time, we were beginning to feel some hope. Kristin was also evaluated for the physical therapy program as an inpatient. At first, she said, "No." She wanted to go home. But as she got to know the therapist who came to her room to evaluate her, she changed her mind. Also, it gave the rest of us a break.

Living in a second-floor apartment had become a problem. Kristin was not able to climb the stairs without a great deal of difficulty. We found an apartment closer to Abby and Gus's home and nearer the hospital. It was also closer to my job. I signed up for family leave. I continued to work almost every day, but there was no problem if I needed time off. The two weeks of inpatient physical therapy were so good for all of us. The IV medication was shrinking the tumor and giving Kristin more movement back in her arm and leg.

Meanwhile, just before moving into the ground floor apartment, Abby's blood work from a routine visit had abnormal results. The tumor marker result had gone up. Explorative surgery was scheduled. This was the same week as our move, and one of Kristin's friends from Michigan was coming to visit. Joanne's visit had been planned several months before these other events occurred.

The move went well. Joanne arrived and stayed for a week, and best of all, the doctor found nothing abnormal. He did many biopsies, and all came back negative for any cancer cells! She was sore and out of commission for some time, but we had a lot to be thankful for.

Kristin continued to require physical therapy after she was discharged home so she went into their outpatient program. We were referred to a company that would transport Kristin to and from MD Anderson. It just amazes me how many genuinely great people were placed in our lives. There were the young men who provided transportation for patients to and from the hospital. They were so kind. If one didn't have the time, then the other one would help us. They even refused to charge us for the last two months of their services.

The physical therapy group at MD Anderson did her final evaluation. It was decided she was at a point where no more improvement would be gained from their services. The brace fitted for her left leg to help her walk was not enough for her to continue walking with her walker. She became more unsteady. We had been using a rented wheelchair, but now she was in her wheelchair most all the time. They ordered a wheelchair measured for her…it was lighter and easier to throw in the trunk.

Abby and Gus would do anything for Kristin. Gus would stop over on his lunch and check on her, or call at any time of the day or night. If Kristin fell and I could not help her up, they would come over any time day or night. A couple of times, we called the fire department. They could help Kristin up so effortlessly and at no charge! Thank the Lord, she never hurt herself.

Her sister was faithful in taking her to support groups at MD Anderson. Even if Kristin didn't want to go, Abby could talk her into going. She stopped in before she went to work on her lunch hour or after work. She loved her sister so much. Every year the MD would provide free tickets to a Houston Astro's game. Kristin and Gus both loved baseball. Abby and I couldn't wait until the games were over! Gus's employer, the microbrewery, held a fundraiser for Kristin.

MD Anderson would often have Lunch and Learn sessions. The support group we would attend was called "The Brain and Spine Group." This session was for the brain support group. I was unable to attend, but Abby planned on picking Kristin up early in the morning. The first fifteen attendants would receive a special gift bag. Abby, of course, wanted a gift bag. She dropped Kristin off in her wheelchair and parked in the parking ramp. Went up to the tenth floor, checked in, and they both received a bag. They went through the line for lunch and finally settled in. The presentation began, however after five minutes, Abby leaned over and asked Kristin, "Do you have spine cancer?" OMG—all that time and effort spent, but what a great story! They enjoyed the meal and left.

When Kristin no longer worked, we were able to get COBRA. It wasn't cheap, but I am very thankful it was an option. Kristin's hospital social worker suggested she apply for Social Security Disability. She told us with Kristin's diagnoses, it would not take long for a decision as to whether she would qualify. I remember saying, "Doesn't that take a long time to go through?" I didn't realize at that time how fast her type of cancer would progress.

Kristin was taking quite a few medications for pain. I remember reassuring her I would not take any of her medications. I leaned heavily on my AA friends. Kristin and I stayed with Bonnie and an AA friend in between our moving to the first-floor apartment. Many times, I would drop Kristin off at Beverly's house while I went to work. Beverly had three dogs to keep her company. She was also mixing up many different "healthy drinks" for Kristin to try. Unfortunately, Kristin said no but yes to Mountain Dew.

This was such a hard time for our family. I remember thinking how thankful I was that my mom had passed away before Abby and Kristin were diagnosed. It would have killed her.

I'll end on a happier note. One of Kristin's last hospitalizations was in a hospital other than MD Anderson. I could navigate quite well in the MD parking ramp because I was familiar with it. I was not familiar with Memorial Herman's parking ramp. Abby and I had met in Kristin's room to visit. She was an inpatient because every time she would stand up, she would pass out. First, they felt she was having seizures when standing, and they gave her anti-seizure medication; that is, until her neurologist placed an electrode on her head, helped stand her up, and she promptly went down. No seizure activity was noted. I felt we lost a lot of time with this misdiagnosis; however, it would not have changed the outcome.

Abby had decided to stay for a bit, and I left for my car. I paid the fee with my credit card just inside the ramp. You would never believe how long I walked on that ramp looking for my car. One level blurred into the next. I thought I was parked between two yellow lines. Every level was a different color. There were eight levels. The more I walked, the more out of control I became. Two hospital employees were smoking, and I'm sure I looked like an Alzheimer's person. My phone was dead, so I could not call security. I finally went back into the hospital up to Kristin's room. I blurted out, "I can't find my car!" They both looked at me like I was nuts.

"Abby, come and help me."

Kristin rolled her eyes and said, "You better help Mom, Abby."

Well, the car was not parked on the yellow level. And it still took some time to drive to the exit. The gate would not go up since I had been there for an additional hour and forty-five minutes. When the guard asked me where I had been, I yelled, "Lost!" He turned around, opened the gate, and never said a word. I know I saw him roll his eyes just like Kristin.

Chapter Twenty

AFTER A COUPLE more days of being an inpatient, it was decided Kristin would come home. Her discharge planner arranged a meeting with a home health company who would spend time with her on the days I would be working. We felt confident they would decide on someone who would be responsible and fill that time with her. I did not request or expect that person to have any other duties than to be with her and help her with any personal needs she might have. I opened the door and greeted her with a good morning. Well, that's all that was necessary for me to realize she was not that person.

She spoke NO ENGLISH, not one word.

I took some time off at the beginning of September. Abby, Gus, and I continued to care for Kristin. The home care agency "Rooms without Walls" continued to visit three times a week. They arranged "field trips" with Kristin. She needed her wheelchair for all transportation by this time. They came to pick her up in a medical minivan. They asked her what interests she had. Baseball was her first response. They visited the Astro's stadium for a behind-the-scenes tour. These outings tired her out, but these were some of the best memories I have of her. She was one of the most fun-loving and positive people I've ever known. No matter what we asked her to do, her response was always, "I'll try."

This is so difficult to write about right now. I'm taking a short "Hallmark movie" break. One of the reasons I sometimes watched Hallmark was simple-minded. The movies always have a happy ending. I know this is simple-minded, a no-brainer, but sometimes that is what I need. Kristin threatened to "block" the channel!

When you look back at a difficult situation you have gone through, you often wonder how you did it. There is no choice to be made. You do one day at a time. I'm not sure how people without faith in a higher power manage situations like this. Not only to get through life here but, more important to me, the life that begins after death. So many of my friends and family back in Michigan continued to send prayers and words of encouragement. Many of her friends came down to visit her. Andrea and Tamara both were life-long friends.

Kristin's second to the last hospital admittance was to manage her pain. She was admitted to MD Anderson, and it was mid-morning when she finally reached her room. The resident who made rounds was someone we had never met. Kristin was not comfortable. The medication ordered was not enough. I called the nurse, asking when to expect the doctor. She told me she had paged him several times, but he had not responded. The nurse said he was finally on her floor and to expect him shortly. The wait was not short. I walked down the hall looking for him. I was on the verge of throwing something at him when he finally entered her room. The light was off, and I sat next to her bedside. The doctor peeked into the dark room, sounding surprised, "You're still here?"

I can't even remember my exact words. It was something like "Why does Kristin have to wait three hours for you to give an order for pain medication?"

He said he wanted to review her chart.

"So, you chose to not talk with her nurse to get a brief report to order one dose of medication?" He stated many of the intense pain medications could cause kidney damage.

I told him I was not aware Kristin's kidneys were failing. They were not, and I knew that. Well, you get the drift of my anger toward him, I'm sure. She was discharged in a couple of days. She was given IV fluids and was more comfortable when we went home. I registered a letter of complaint with the hospital and received an email and phone call. I told them we were very satisfied with MD Anderson except for this incident, which was unacceptable.

Her last admittance began with Kristin waking up, frightened and telling me she could not see. She had lost the vision in one eye when she was three from NF. But now, the pupil in the other eye was dilated. I called 911, and Kristin was transported to MD Anderson's emergency room. The MRI showed cancer had spread to her optic nerve and audio nerves. There was also more growth in her brain stem, as well as in her spinal fluid. The medical diagnosis was listed as Leptomeningeal. I think I said something like, "so, what do we do now?'

The doctor walked Abby and me into another room. She proceeded to tell us there was no more that could be done. I knew she was going to say that.

"We want her to be as comfortable as possible."

She was admitted to the same floor she always went to. We stayed with her that night. The next day was Monday. Gus, Abby, and I met her social worker to arrange for hospice to help care for her at home. Her pain meds were to be given every four hours as needed. We rang for the nurse every four hours if they were late.

I knew that pain medication could suppress her breathing, but I knew she needed them for comfort. Then as I looked at her, I realized she wasn't breathing.

"Abby, I don't think she is breathing."

Abby opened the door and went running down the hall, "My sister's not breathing, my sister's not breathing!" And that was it…

We had a celebration service in Michigan at the church we grew up in, South Blendon Reformed. We encouraged people to wear sports T-shirts of Kristin's favorite teams, the White Sox and Da Bears. Everyone shared stories. It was a sweet time of reflection.

One of my best friends from AA loves baseball; we call him Baseball Mike. He worked with Abby, and in the spring, twelve of Kristin's best friends and family went to the White Sox Stadium and spread her ashes along the first baseline.

She would have loved it...

In looking back whenever Kristin and I would have a difficult day I would say to her, "Honey, this day wasn't so bad. I'm still sober."

Early in my recovery, I loved reading "The Promises." Two of my favorites are: "We will know a new freedom and a new happiness," and "We will intuitively know how to handle situations which used to baffle us."

I knew if I wanted to stay sober, I had to want something more than drinking. The desire to drink gradually grew weaker, and with the help of my higher power, it has disappeared... Despite life's many challenges, I am grateful I do not need to depend on drugs or alcohol to get me through.

Today, now thanks to having had a "last call" for good, my final calling is to embrace sobriety and live life to the fullest, regardless of any obstacles I may face.

I love being sober!

Family Photo Album

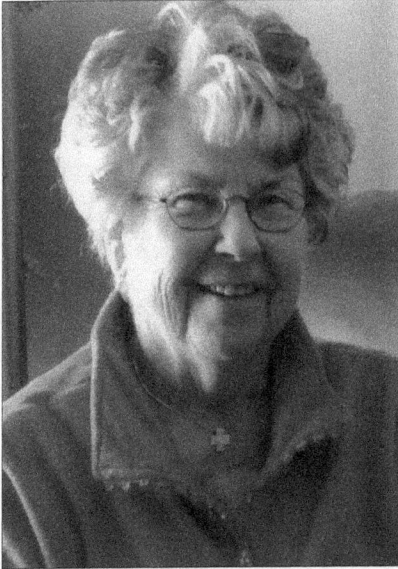

Mom, Marie, She never gave up
on me!

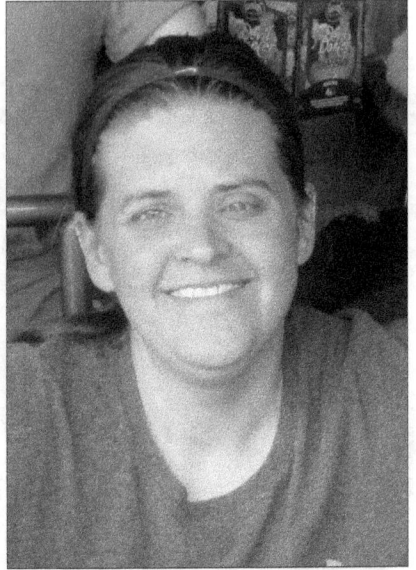

Kristin Joy Lillie.

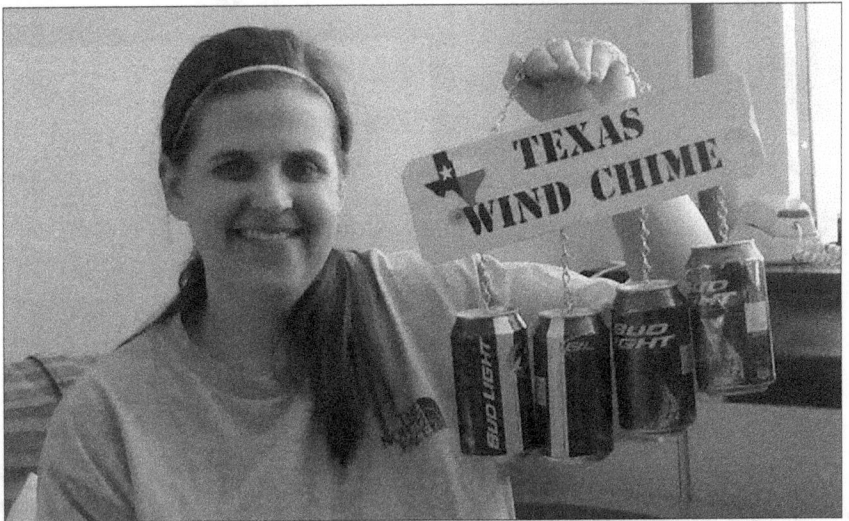

Kristen with Texas wind chimes.

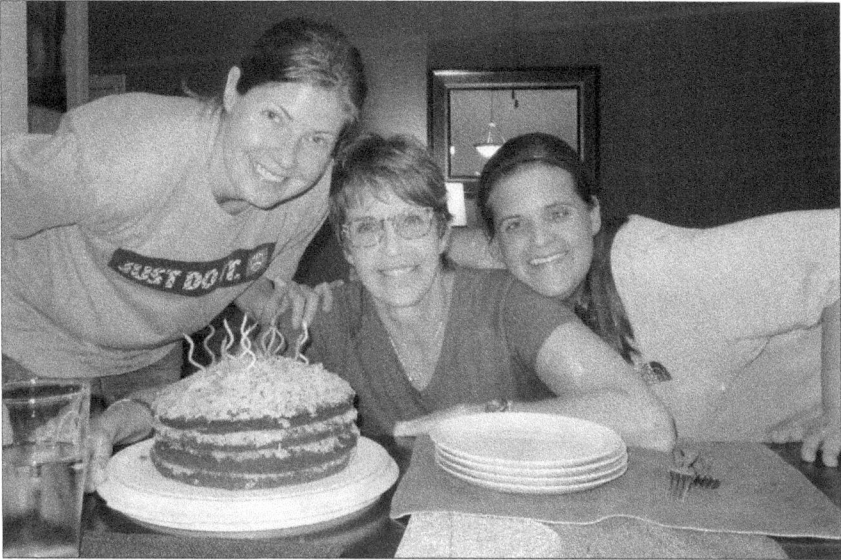

Sarah, Mom, Kristin—Just moved to Houston and celebrating Mom's birthday.

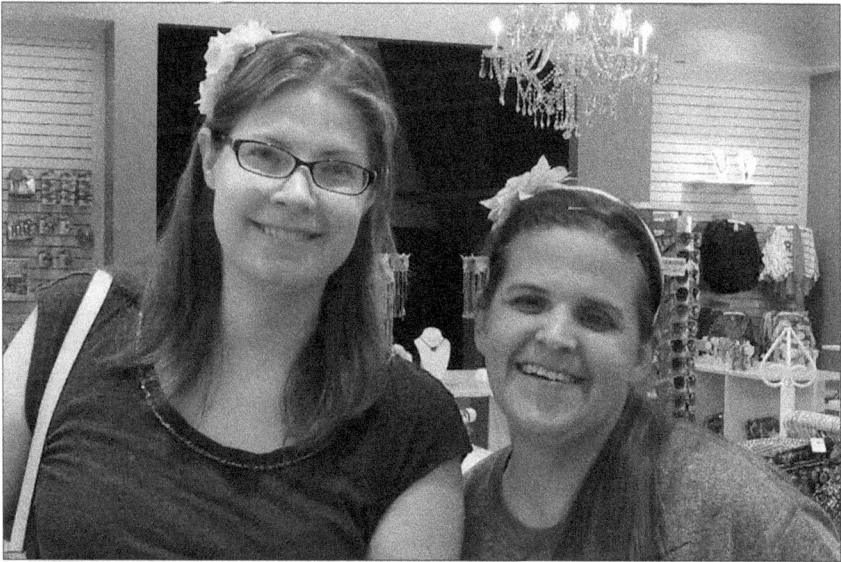

Just moved to Houston and doing a little shopping.

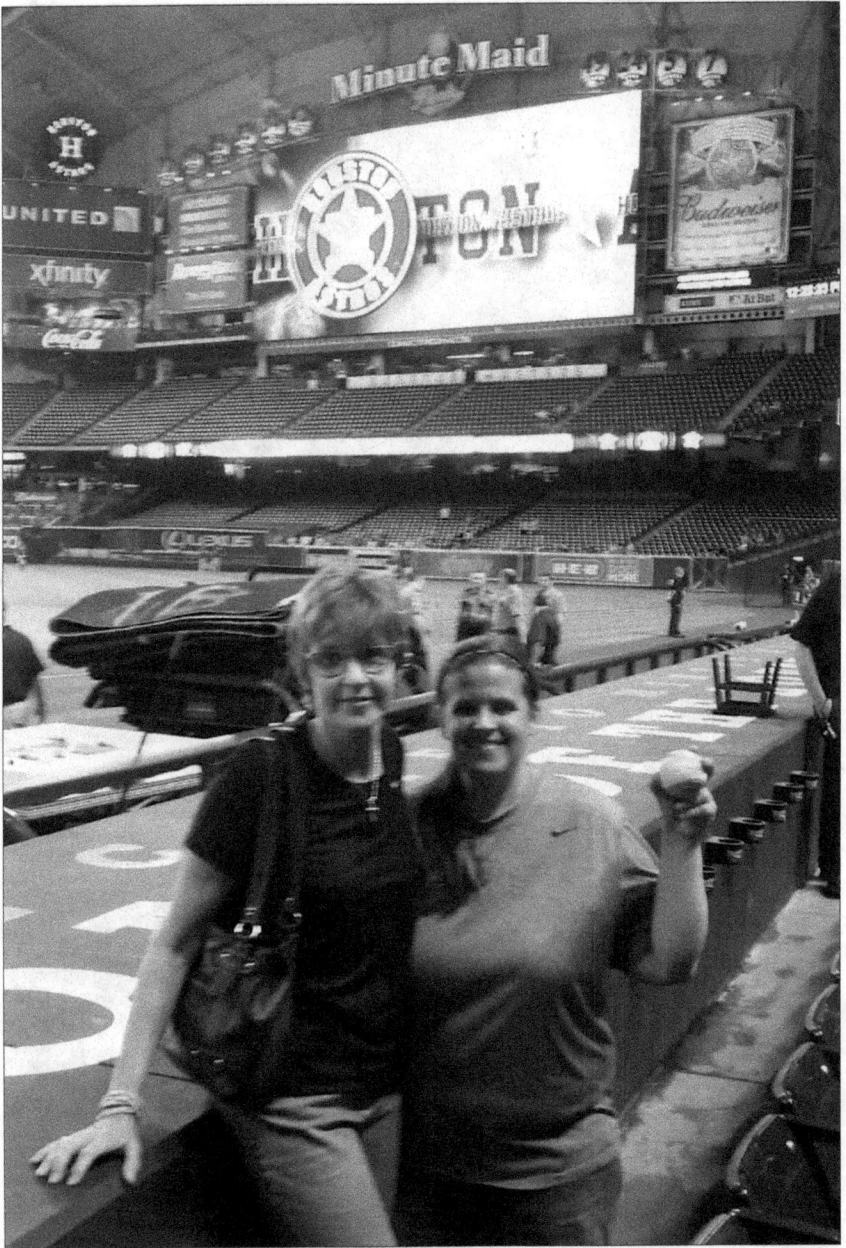

Kristin and Mom at a Houston Astros Game courtesy of Baseball Mike.

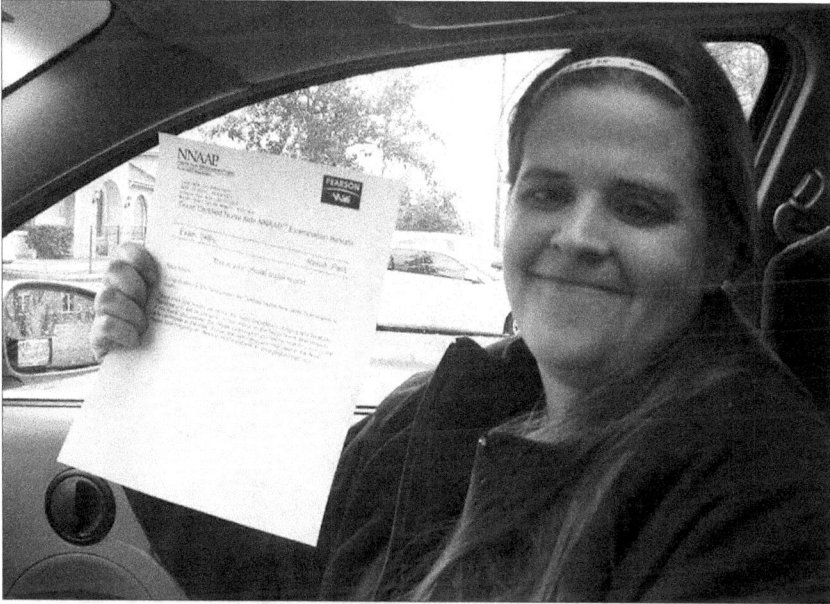

Kristin's graduation for her CNA-Certified Nursing Assistant!!

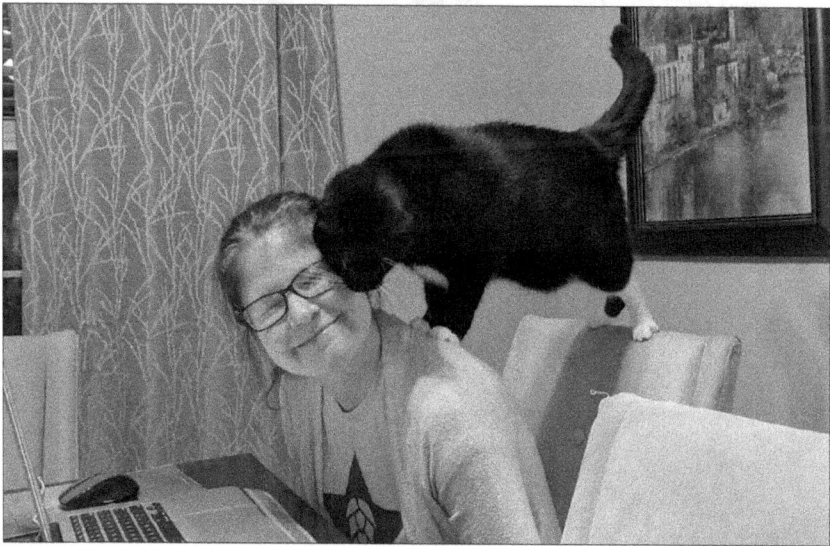

Sarah and Dale.

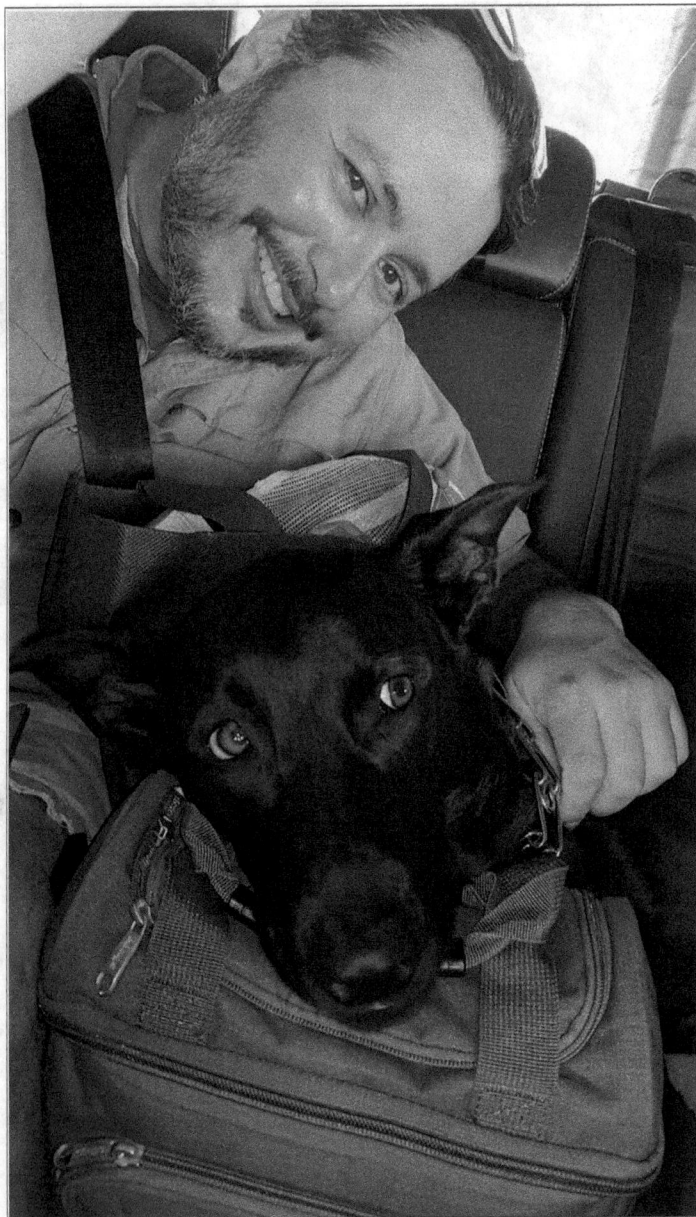

Gus—the best son-in-law ever, and sweet Luna Joy

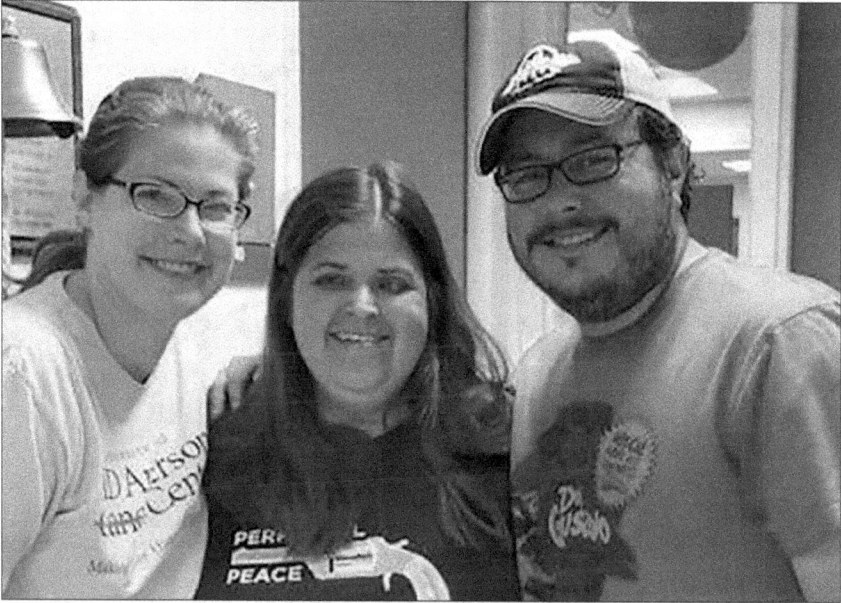

Finishing Radiation Therapy

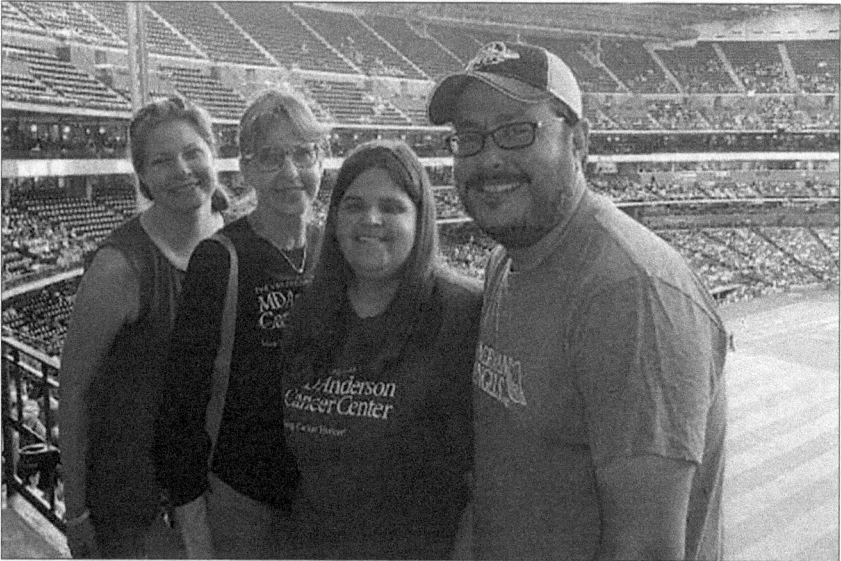

Houston Astros Game. Compliments of MD Anderson Cancer Center.

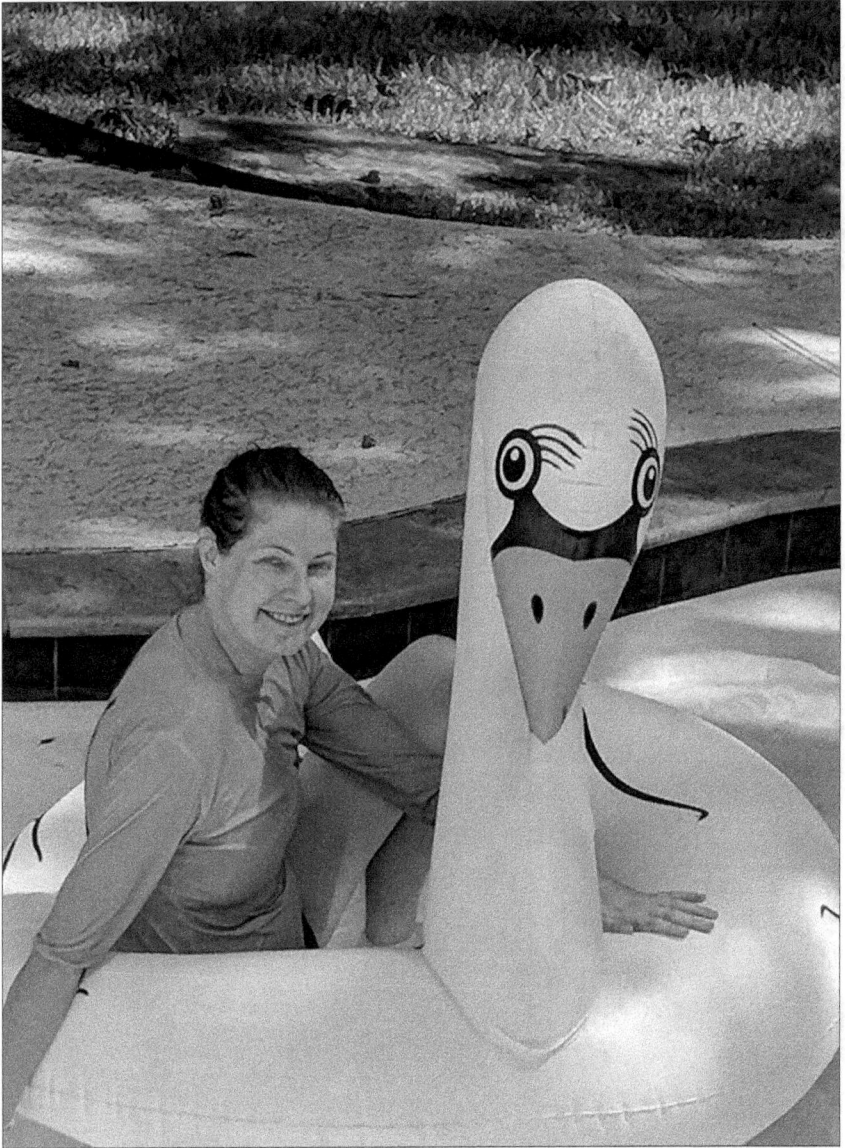

Sarah and Kristin swimming. As Kristin lost more movement of her right side due to the tumor growth, we all enjoyed swimming in Gus and Sarah's pool.

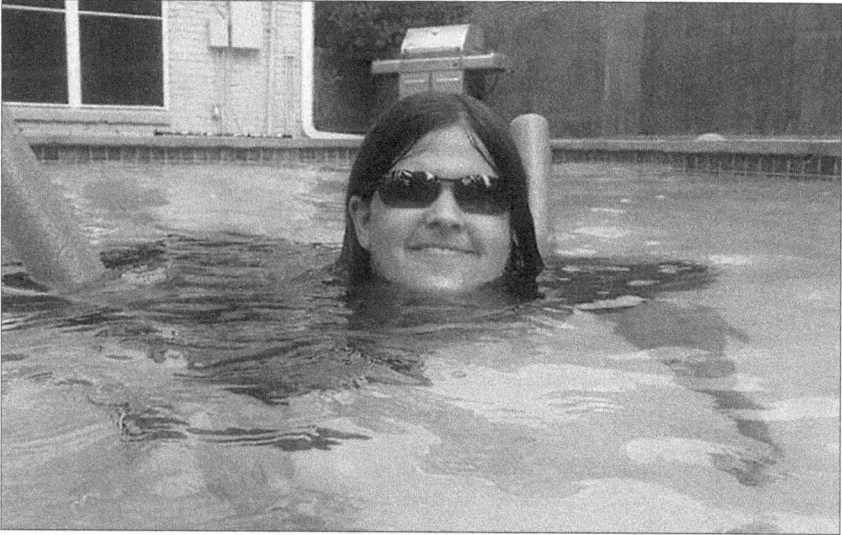

Kristin in the pool Summer of 2015.

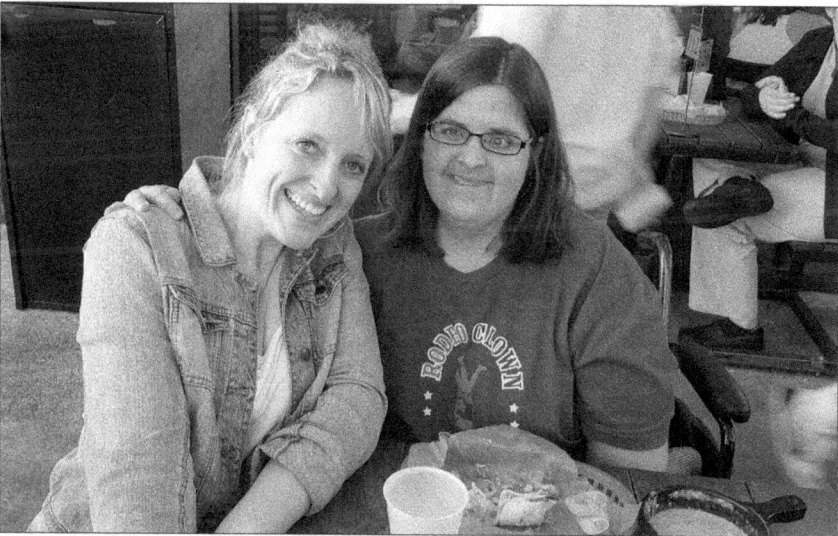

Kristin and Andrea—a friend from Michigan visiting and eating at her favorite taco restaurant.

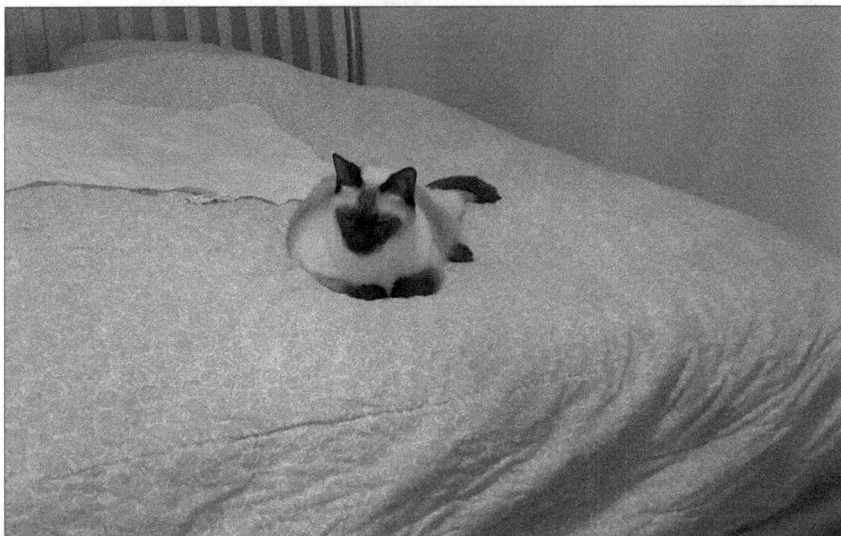

Max waiting for Kristin to come to bed—every night.

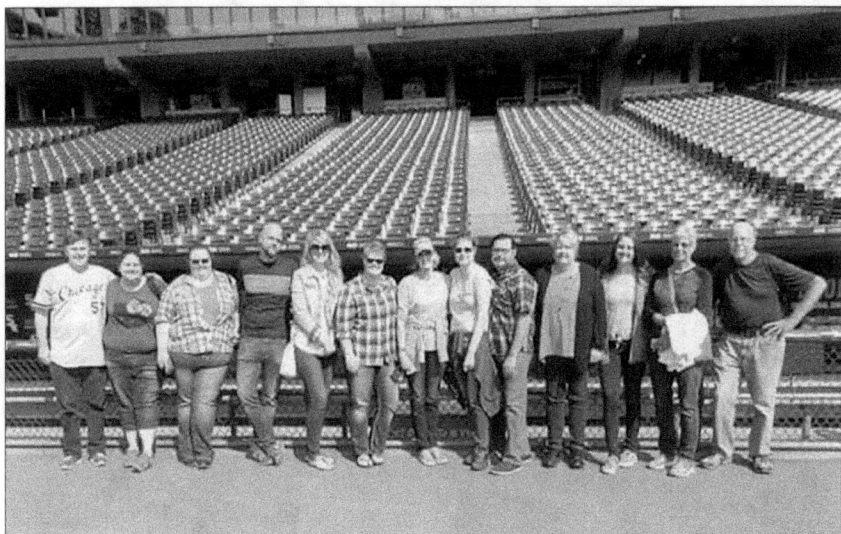

Family and friends spreading Kristin's ashes at the White Sox Stadium. Her favorite team. We know she would have loved it.

www.ingramcontent.com/pod-product-compliance
Lightning Source LLC
Chambersburg PA
CBHW052136270326
41930CB00012B/2905